# Meal Prep

# for

# Weight Loss

New ways for weekly meal prep and healthy meal prep, develop your diet meal plan for weight loss with a right food strategy

**Amanda Davis**

## Text Copyright © [Leanne Paradox]

## Legal & Disclaimer

The information contained in this book and its contents is not designed to replace or take the place of any form of medical or professional advice; and is not meant to replace the need for independent medical, financial, legal or other professional advice or services, as may be required. The content and information in this book has been provided for educational and entertainment purposes only.

The content and information contained in this book has been compiled from sources deemed reliable, and it is accurate to the best of the Author's knowledge, information and belief. However, the Author cannot guarantee its accuracy and validity and cannot be held liable for any errors and/or omissions. Further, changes are periodically made to this book as and when needed. Where appropriate and/or necessary, you must consult a professional (including but not limited to your doctor, attorney, financial advisor or such other professional advisor) before using any of the suggested remedies, techniques, or information in this book.

Upon using the contents and information contained in this book, you agree to hold harmless the Author from and against any damages, costs, and expenses, including any legal fees potentially resulting from the application of any of the information provided by this book. This disclaimer applies to any loss, damages or injury caused by the use and application, whether directly or indirectly, of any advice or information presented, whether for breach of contract, tort, negligence, personal injury, criminal intent, or under any other cause of action.

You agree to accept all risks of using the information presented inside this book.

You agree that by continuing to read this book, where appropriate and/or necessary, you shall consult a professional (including but not limited to your doctor, attorney, or financial advisor or such other advisor as needed) before using any of the suggested remedies, techniques, or information in this book.

# Table of Contents

# Introduction

Meal preppers, welcome! If you have a goal to lose weight and trim down, you've started at the right place as meal prepping can really help you to reach your goals. There's something about being organized and dedicated which makes you really want to stick to your goals and eat the foods you know will deliver you to your healthiest weight yet.

These recipes are not "diet" recipes; they are healthy, nutritious, filling, and tasty recipes. I don't believe you need to cut out food groups or deprive yourself in order to lose weight. In fact, eating properly, eating enough, and eating foods that satisfy you will result in weight loss you can maintain and sustain. So, if you're looking for a particular diet or eating style, then this might not be the book for you! But I hope it is, as I know you'll love these recipes as much as I do.

Oh, I should add a bit about me! I am not a nutritionist or dietitian. But I am someone who has successfully lost weight through sensible and healthy eating, and of course, meal prepping! I want to pass on my recipes and my knowledge of meal prepping so you too can experience the same success and health benefits.

Please consult your doctor or nutritionist for advice and guidance if you are looking to lose large amounts of weight, or if you have health issues which might be affected due to a change in diet. This book is a friendly and supportive guideline to help you lose weight in a healthy way, without extreme changes or deprivation.

Now, let's get into the ins and outs of meal prepping!

# Chapter 1

# What Is Meal Prep?

Meal prepping is the art of preparing your meals the night (or a few nights) before eating. It usually involves preparing a few portions of each meal, packing them away in airtight containers, and storing in the fridge. Many people prep their meals these days, because it saves time, encourages healthy eating, and controls portions. Sometimes, the meal is completely prepared and cooked in its entirety before being stacked away in the fridge or freezer until it is needed. Whereas sometimes, meals are only partially prepared so they can be cooked right before eating. For example, you can prep lasagna by cooking the sauces and layering it all up before covering and storing in the fridge, raw. You would then place the lasagna into a preheated oven before eating the next night. Whatever prepping method you choose, it's a great way to manage your time and your diet!

Meal prepping is a new concept for busy cooks to help them plan the week with pre-planned meals and quick access to the Ingredients.

Everybody has schedule overload these days, especially if you work full-time, kids to take to school, home from school, soccer and theatre practice, after hours work obligations, meals to cook and a house to clean.

Don't you feel overwhelmed and tired already?

The basics of meal-prep works like this.

You plan the menus for the week for breakfast, lunch, and supper. Add snacks if you wish, we have plenty listed in the last chapter.

You make the list of Ingredients for the week.

You buy the Ingredients and the proper storage containers.

You cook everything on one afternoon, usually in two hours or less.

You refrigerate and freeze the contents, labeling each packet.

When you are ready to eat, you heat them and serve them.

You have just eliminated at least six hours of work a week, and decreased spending, and stayed on your high protein, low carb diet.

Hurray! Victory!

Benefits of Meal-Prepping

At first, meal prepping may seem like a lot of work that takes up a weekend afternoon, very precious time in my household. There are so many exciting benefits of meal-prepping I'm not quite sure where to start. Here are a few for your consideration:

Your kitchen time will be cut by as much as 75 percent, once you get the hang of it and make it a personal habit.

Your grocery bill will instantly drop.  One of the reasons is because you are buying in bulk and all at one time. Another of the reasons is the impulse factor. Have you ever gone to the grocery store for just one item and came home with a trunk load of many unnecessary purchases, all because you were hungry?

Using the concepts of meal prep allows you to know what you are eating with the correct portion size. Eating out is too much a temptation to buy the wrong dinner choices, and eating leftovers so you don't have to store them is still overeating.

With the extra time you gain from eating properly and preparing your meals once a week, you can now add the exercise plan to your day that you've always wanted to start, but never had enough time.

The Helpful Equipment

 Note this equipment is helpful, but not a necessity. Everything can be cooked on a stove, using a skillet, or pots and pans. Knives can be used to cut and plates can function as cutting boards. However, since the point of meal-prep is to save both time and money, these appliances pay for themselves in many ways.

A Crock-pot

This ageless appliance lets you cook and rest at the same time. Although there are only a few crock-pot recipes within these covers, these will not be the only recipes you prepare. If you use a crockpot on cooking day, you can use a larger and less expensive cut of meat. This can be a real savings.

Skillets that are oven proof and non-stick

Most likely if you cook any meals ever you have a skillet or two. In this cookbook, we strive to mess up less dishes. Some of the recipes require browning and then baking. An ovenproof skillet can do both, eliminating one more dish to wash.

At least 3 mixing bowls in large, medium and small sizes

It may be likely that you have these, but not everyone does. As you double or triple recipes when you cook, you will need more than one size and more than one in quantity.

A Blender

Some soups taste better when blended to a creamy puree. It is always easier and tastier to emulsify salad dressings, instead of whipping them by hand in a bowl. You do not have to buy an expensive model as 5 or 6 settings will be enough for the blending instructions we have included.

A Food Processor

When you are preparing multiple meals, using a food processor to chop, slice, and dice saves so much energy and time. The foods are also healthier. Did you know that purchased shredded cheese can include 10 percent wood pulp, commonly called saw dust? When you are purchasing 10 pounds of cheese, you are receiving eight pounds of cheese and two pounds of sawdust. What's more, you are eating it! Save your health by shredding your own blocks of cheese with the food processor. You can freeze it for later use and know the contents of what you are eating.

Good quality sharp knives

Sharp knives make cutting faster and help to keep you from cutting yourself by pressing too hard.

Cutting Boards

Cutting Boards come in several materials and sizes. They protect surfaces and allow the air to circulate underneath while the baked goods cool.

Keep in mind that the construction materials of a cutting board will determine its cleanliness. For example:

Bamboo cutting boards are self-healing. This allows the cuts made by knives to heal on their own. The bamboo cutting boards are very good to knives as they do not dull them quickly. Bamboo is a porous material, which allows bacteria to seep into the cuts. Even disinfecting promptly after use will never eliminate the germs that have accumulated on a wood cutting board.

Glass canning jars with lids, pint sized and quart sized

One of the lesser known secrets is that salad stored in a Ball or Mason jar with a tight sealing lid will stay fresh in the refrigerator for seven full days! This makes the dinner salad, stored in a quart jar, easy to place into serving plates. Salads stored in pint jars are perfect for toting in the thermal lunch bag for a healthy lunch. The salad dressing can be included in the jar and will still be fresh.

Foil containers

These can be expensive, but dollar stores have these priced better than grocery stores. Buy the containers that include lids, baking sizes and the individual sizes.

Plastic containers

Use the food prep containers that are custom designed for Meal-prep. These have no BPAs, are apportioned in the right serving sizes, and are inexpensive. They are dishwasher safe, freezer safe, and can be used in the microwave. Buy enough containers for all your family members to eat three meals a day for one week. You will also need zip-lock freezer bags, pint-sized and snack-sized. Using leftover whipped topping bowls or margarine containers can be less expensive, but they are not constructed to be heated in the microwave or stored for long-term in the freezer.

# Chapter 2

# Macronutrients And Healthy Food

The macronutrients that constitute our diet are:

The Carbohydrates: also called carbon carbohydrates, sugars or more commonly, are the primary source of energy. They also contain the fibers, which we will define a little later.

The Fat: fatty acids also called "fat" or fat are molecules that form the organic fat. They play an important role in the constitution of cell membranes, energy production, and body temperature and more generally in the metabolism of the human being.

The Proteins: they are essential molecules for the life of cells and the constitution of human tissues (muscles, hair, skin, etc.).

Macronutrients are molecules that provide energy to our body or that participate directly or indirectly in metabolism. They are called "macro" in order to differentiate them from micronutrients such as vitamins, minerals, enzymes, etc.

Carbohydrates

It is the main source of energy of the body.

As you have guessed, it's about sugars, and yes sugars, we'll always need them. Everything depends then which sugars to privilege, and there, it becomes more complicated.

In theory, these are the complex sugars to favor at the expense of simple sugars, but that does not help you much!

What are the foods based on complex sugars and those based on simple sugars?

Simple sugars have a high glycemic index (Glucose and sucrose ...) they are present in sweets, pastries, classic white sugar, in many prepared dishes, sauces (ketchup, bbq sauce, sweet and sour)

Complex sugars, meanwhile, have a low glycemic index; they are present in cereals (whole grains, attention!) and legumes.

Sugar in fruits is also an excellent source of energy, but we must not forget that fructose must first be treated in the liver before 'be used by the body, and it cannot be part of the complex sugars, it is a so-called fast sugar, but does not have a too high glycemic index, (IG: 20 against 100 for glucose), which differentiates it especially glucose classic is that the carbohydrate intake is supplemented with a contribution of fiber, minerals and vitamins.

## THE PROTIDES

In common parlance we often tend to call them "proteins", but this is an abuse of language, and yes, in fact the protides is a sort of "family" grouping proteins, amino acids, and peptides.

When we talk about proteins "protiderotides" we immediately think of our muscles, and yes you know well they are made up, but we must not forget that they are also made of 70% water, moreover the water content of our body represents on average about 65% of our mass, small parenthesis

Back to our proteins, except the muscles (myosin, actin, myoglobin) , they are also present in our hair, nail our skin (keratin), but also in our red blood cells (globin).

They provide a multitude of functions within the cells:

Cell renewal

Role of protection (hair, nails, skin)

Physiological functioning (information transmission, digestion, immune defense)

Secondary energy role (after carbohydrates)

and it is also our only source of nitrogen (essential for life) , and yes it is a present element to link amino acids to each other.

Proteins are of animal or vegetable origin (legumes, cereals)

Contrary to many received ideas, vegetable proteins are not of less good quality than animal proteins, on the contrary.

Indeed, animal proteins also contain so-called saturated fats (we'll talk about it later), favoring weight gain, cardiovascular risks and clot formation, on the contrary vegetable proteins are rich in fibers without any saturated fat.

**LIPIDS**

Despite their demonization, it is a primordial macro nutrient essential to our proper functioning.

Lipids are an important energy store, they are essential to regulate the temperature of our body, and very importantly, they are one of the major constituents of membranes    and the nervous system, indeed lipids surround and strengthen our lymph.

On the other hand, lipids are not all of the same quality!

This is where the difference, always and again, good and bad fats, so we distinguish different types of fatty acids: saturated, monounsaturated or polyunsaturated.

The saturated = to limit! They increase the cardiovascular risk as stated above (contained in fatty meats, sausages, butter or cream, vegetable fats biscuits and industrial dishes)

Mono-unsaturated = also called omega-9 contained in oilseeds (almonds, hazelnuts, walnuts ...) and avocado

Poly-unsaturated = these are omega 6 and 3, these are essential fatty acids, our body is unable to synthesize them, they contribute to the proper functioning of our cardiovascular system, some studies have demonstrated that omega-3 fatty acids promote lipolysis (provision of fat to provide energy to the body) it is not beautiful, so do not hesitate to consume virgin oils first cold pressed (olive oil, rapeseed),also in oily fish, but I cannot encourage you to consume since they too often contain heavy metals such as mercury, and especially for our biodiversity and ethics, it is better to leave them there where he is, it was the little ethical parenthesis

An individual's macros are calculated as a percentage of the total calories consumed. "So, for example, if you are an active middle-aged and 60k-weight individual who goes to the gym regularly and follow a 1600-calorie diet, you need 40% of your calories to come from carbohydrates, 30% of proteins and 30% of fats.

These proportions would be normal for those who do not train for a living, or for people who are active, but not for endurance athletes. This is what those calculations would look like:

1600 x 0.40 = 640 calories from carbohydrates

1600 x 0.30 = 480 calories of protein

1600 x 0.30 = 480 calories from fat

"To convert those calories figures into grams, carbohydrates and proteins are divided by 4, because both carbohydrates and proteins provide 4 calories per gram, "and fat by 9, because fat contributes 9 calories. per gram. " This is how those calculations would work:

640/4 = 160 grams of carbohydrates

480/4 = 120 grams of protein

480/9 = 53 grams of fat

The proportion of macros will change according to your objectives. "It is important to take into account your level of activity and the type of exercises you do,

For example, if you are strength training you will need to increase your protein intake to facilitate muscle recovery and prevent injuries. While if you focus more on cardio, you will have to increase carbohydrates to prevent the wear of glycogen stores.

## WHAT IS THE EASIEST WAY TO CALCULATE YOUR OWN MACROS?

When entering your data in an online macro calculator: age, height, weight, sex, activity level, target weight, frequency and intensity with which you lift weights. If It Fits Your Macros, which also asks when you want to achieve your goals, or Healthy Eater , which is simpler, but produces similar calculations.

## *The Benefits Of Counting Macros*

It's about getting the right amount of each one right, so as not to fall short or exceed your body's needs. By achieving that balance, your body will function at its highest level and you will recover properly. It also activates other systems such as immune, digestive and sleep.

"It's like a group of workers in which everyone does their job so that the whole body works at its maximum performance.

It is clear that this "work" depends on your level of activity and your objectives. "If you are an athlete, macros are very important. Also, if you eat adjusting to your macros, you don't have to eliminate any important food groups or deprive yourself of anything.

But if you want to lose fat, gain muscle, it is very important to consider the source and quality of the food you eat. "I have seen people who count macros stuffing themselves with donuts because 'it fits their macros', but they perform less and feel worse than if they had opted for sweet potatoes or other types of carbohydrates," he adds.

## THE BAD THING ABOUT COUNTING MACROS

In an IIFYM diet, the important thing is not to deprive yourself of something, but to feed you so that your body functions in the most effective way. But counting macros can take time. Not only do you have to know the proportions, but you also have to measure food on an appropriate scale. So if you feel lazy to weigh everything you eat, counting macros is not made for you.

In addition, monitoring, tracking and weighing everything you eat can create an unhealthy relationship with food. Anytime the numbers go up and you like to control your diet. But if you have suffered eating disorders in the past, counting macros is probably not a good idea.

Like any other diet, counting macros is not a panacea. It can help you make the body function very effectively, and even serve you to reach certain goals, but remember that the most important thing is the quality of what you eat. As an athlete, you know that diet is only part of the equation, so the best is what best suits your lifestyle and, therefore, you manage to maintain in the long term.

# Chapter 3

# Success In Meal Prepping

Utilize the freezer

Frozen prepped meals are a lifesaver during busy and chaotic times. A good way to utilize the freezer is to double the recipe for a particular meal and put half of the servings in the fridge for the consequent days, and put the other half in the freezer for later down the track. You'll be very pleased you did so, especially during times when your meal-prep game schedule is slipping!

Keep your macros in mind: proteins, carbs, fats

You don't want to sit down to your prepped lunch only to find that it's too filling or not filling enough due to unbalanced macros. Remember to include a portion of protein, some good fats, and some healthy wholegrain carbs for optimum energy and satiety. Most of the recipes in this book have a great balance of macros, but you can adjust them to suit your needs and preferences.

Stock-up on flavor-packing non-perishables

Herbs, spices, vinegars, oils, and natural flavorings can turn any simple dish into a tasty masterpiece, with very little added calories. What's more, they last a very long time in the pantry so you don't need to worry about using them up before their best-before date. Splash out on a big haul of natural, flavor-giving Ingredients to pack into your meal-prep box. This means that you can use simple base Ingredients, and adjust the flavors with the addition of healthy and low-cal seasonings.

Invest in storage equipment

This is an important one. To successfully prep, you need containers to store your meals in. High-quality plastic or glass containers with airtight lids are ideal, especially if you can find a set which includes different sizes. Small, single-serve containers are really handy for breakfasts such as oats and chia pudding, and snacks such as fruit and nut mix. Pyrex bowls which have airtight lids are ideal for large salads and soups. Have a shop around and find yourself a few value packs, and allocate a special box, drawer, or cupboard, especially for your meal-prep containers.

Get creative with color

During my own meal prepping journey I found that using bright and varied colors really helped me to get excited about making, and eating my prepped meals. A pile of red cabbage with bright red bell peppers and some vibrant green cilantro – beautiful! Rich yellow corn kernels, inky black beans, glossy red chili, and pale green avocado, it looks as amazing as it tastes. If you're like me, then you'll get a kick out of putting together beautiful and fresh-looking meals to fill your containers. Fresh fruits, veggies, herbs, and rich spices are the best sources of edible color.

Predict your cravings and prep accordingly

If you don't feel like eating a particular meal, then don't prep it. Don't think that you must eat a certain type of dish simply because it seems like the healthiest option. You can make any dish healthy! Even if it's traditionally a junk food. For example, you will find recipes for burgers and rich pastas in this book, but they are nutritious versions which fit in with your weight loss plans. If you've got a craving for sweeter dishes, then try a yummy oatmeal with dates for breakfast! If you feel like something a bit heavier for dinner (tiredness, hormones, and overindulgence can make us crave comfort foods) then choose a recipe for dinner with sweet potatoes and beans to fill you up. The bottom line? Prep foods you want to eat that particular week! This way, you'll avoid seeking other foods or snacks to satisfy you in between meals.

Make a plan and stick to it

This is where you need to be a bit strict and structured. Decide on a day to complete your prepping, set the time aside, and stick to it. Get your shopping done on the same day so your produce and meats are fresh, then set aside a couple of hours to prep, prep, prep! If you end up missing a prep day and you don't have the time to make up for it, you might find you slip back into day-to-day meals and the unhealthy choices and unbalanced portion sizes may creep back. Once the routine has been established it will be so easy!

Make it fun

Cooking should be as fun as eating, in my opinion! And the same goes for prepping. If you enjoy yourself, you'll get into a positive mindset about meal prepping, and a positive mindset about food will follow on. There are many ways to make meal-prep sessions fun! Play music, have a glass of wine, watch your favorite TV show, anything that relaxes you and puts you at ease as you work. Weight loss needn't be a drag, it can actually be an enjoyable and nourishing experience if you make the process work in a way that you enjoy.

# Chapter 4

# Diet Meal Planning

By planning your meals in advance, you're able to buy in bulk which will save you money. You can usually store a meal for at least two weeks in the freezer too. It can help you save money at lunchtime too when you have prepped leftovers.

Weight Loss

The ketogenic diet already helps you to lose weight but planning your meals in advance will help you to save a little more cash too. With meal planning, you know exactly how much you're going to eat at a time, which can help to keep you from overeating.

A meal routine will also make it easier to know how many net carbs you're putting in your body each day. You can even label the meals with the amount of net carbs in each one.

Easy Grocery Shopping

It's easy to go grocery shopping when you know exactly what you'll be eating and when. Make a list, and just get everything off it. If you are prepping your snacks too, you don't even have to deviate off the list for everything you need.

Just divide your shopping list into different categories like fruits, protein, frozen food, etc., and it'll be easier than ever to avoid aisles where you'd spend too much money or end up straying from the ketogenic diet.

Less Waste

Most of the time, you can just eat out of the dish that you've stored your food in. this helps you to cut down on paper plates, plastic utensils, and will keep you from wasting your food if you've prepped in advance. You unitize all the Ingredients that you bought during the week, and it helps you to plan accordingly.

Time Saver

This is the main reason that people decide to start meal prepping. It's hard to find time to cook three meals a day, but that's exactly what the ketogenic diet requires. By saving time when cooking, you're less likely to eat junk food or fast food too.

Stress Reduction

Stress can affect your digestive system, disrupt your sleep and even cause your immune system to suffer. It can be hard to come home from a long day of work and then pan for dinner. With meal prep, you have a dedicated day to get the dinners ready, which allows you to relax most of the time.

How to Start Prepping Today

Let's

look at everything you need to start meal prepping today. There are certain Ingredients you'll need as well as equipment to get started with.

Meal Prepping Equipment

You'll find essential equipment and what it's used for below.

- Cutting Board: You should try to get boards made from solid materials because they're corrosion resistant and non-porous which makes them easier to clean than wood or bamboo boards. Try plastic, glass, or even marble cutting boards for easier clean up.

- Measuring Cups: It's important that you measure out your spices and condiments accurately.

- Measuring Spoons: Even when you're prepping in bulk, you may still only need a small amount of some spices.

- Glass Bows: Glass bowls are considered easier, but nonmetallic containers will also be needed for storing meat and marinades.

- Packaging Materials: Your non-metallic containers and glass bowls will be important for this as well, but you may also want bento boxes that are freezer safe or even Tupperware. Make sure that you have freezer safe containers too.

- Paper Towels & Kitchen Towels: These will be required for draining meat.

- Knives: Your knives should be sharp to slice meat accordingly. Remember to cut away from your body, and you should wash your knives while cutting different food types

- Kitchen Scale: A kitchen scale can make some recipes much easier, allowing for much more accurate measurements.

- Internal Thermometer: You'll need to check the internal temperature of many meats, especially if you're making snacks like jerky.

- Baking Sheet: This will be needed for many recipes, especially sheet cakes, cookies, or even jerky.

- Colander: You'll have to drain some vegetables and rices.

- Skillets & Pans: It's going to be easier to cook if you have the right sized pan or skillet for what you're doing. You'll need baking dishes too!

Stocking Your Kitchen

While it's impossible to give you a list of each ingredient you'll ever use, there are some basics that you'll want to keep on hand. Before you start prepping for the week, make a comprehensive shopping list according to your meal plan.

- Cupboard Ingredients: Sea Salt, Black Pepper, Tomato Sauce, Tomato Paste, Crushed Tomatoes, Garlic Powder, Onion Powder, Ground Spices, Powdered Sweeteners, Liquid Sweeteners, Canned Vegetables, Almond Flour, Coconut Oil, Coconut Milk, Desiccated Coconut, Nuts & Seeds, Olive Oil, Balsamic Vinegar, White Wine Vinegar.

- Vegetables: Avocado, Onions, Fresh Garlic, Zucchini.

- Fridge: A Pound of Butter, Cream, Yogurt, Eggs, Baby Carrots, Cherry Tomatoes.

Simple Steps for Meal Prep

For whatever day you get started, you're going to want to streamline the process as much as possible. To do that, just follow the simple steps below to help you get started.

Step 1: Make a Shopping List

You'll want to make a shopping list the day before for best results. In the beginning of your 21-day plan, you'll need to make it for a few short days, but at the end, your shopping list will be for a week at a time. Expect to dedicate most of the day to meal prep but remember that it will make life easier.

Step 2: Go Shopping

You'll want to go in and get out when it comes to the grocery store so that you aren't tempted by unhealthy snacks that will pull you out of ketosis. If you have mostly vegetables, try going to the local farmers market where there's less temptation too. A butcher's shop for your meat can also help.

Step 3: Start with a Clean Area

It's going to be easier to start cooking if you clean your area beforehand, and make sure that you have your containers clean too. It's important to make sure you have everything on hand, and it'll help to make it all go by a little quicker.

Step 4: Start Cooking!

Now the only thing left is to start cooking, but make sure that you let your food completely cool before packing it up. If you don't let your food cool, then you can ruin the texture and it may become soggy upon reheating.

Ketogenic diet is not one of those fad diets that you have probably used before, this diet is completely different because it does not put you in a "fast" or "calorie deprivation" mode, rather it works by simply switching your body's mechanism from the usual high carb reliant to a fat-burning mode – this mode makes it easier for your body to build more muscles and cut down fat deposit.

Contrary to the beliefs in some quarters that Low carb Ketogenic diet will cause high fat deposits in the body, due to the presence of low carbs and high protein and fat contents, the reverse is completely the case. The "Low carb" rule here does not mean you have to consume excess saturated fats that cause high cholesterol, it simply allows you to lower your carb supplies enough, and increase other components marginally. The main benefit of Ketogenic diet is that it forces the body to rely on stored fat and fat from diet, as the primary source of energy.

Ketogenic diet helps build more lean muscles while losing fat. The main reason for this is that individuals placed on Ketogenic diets have been found to force their bodies to use up more water, and secondly, the lowered Insulin hormones will force the kidneys to remove excess Sodium and the combined effect of these is that there is a speedy loss of weight within the shortest possible period of time.

Another benefit of Ketogenic diet is that, it targets fat deposit in the most difficult parts of the body, most especially the abdominal region, thighs and the upper chest areas. Starving yourself may not help cut fat in the most difficult regions, even when you lose fat in such areas, they may return quickly, but this is not the case with Ketogenic diets. Losing weight around your mid-section and around vital organs is necessary in order to avoid serious fat-related diseases.

Ketogenic diets increases the amount of HDL cholesterols while reducing LDL cholesterol levels. Choosing the right type of unsaturated fats in your Ketogenic diet will help increase good cholesterols (HDL cholesterols), and these are healthy for the heart and general wellbeing. Ketogenic diets also help regulate blood sugar levels while reducing the risks of insulin intolerance. When carbs are broken down, they release  sugar into the blood quickly and this increases blood sugar rapidly, a condition that triggers more supply of Insulin hormones, but when Ketogenic diets replace high carb diets, less sugar are released slowly into the body, a situation that can stabilize the secretion of Insulin hormones.

# Chapter 5

# Shopping List

When shopping applies: Well-planned is usually already won. Anyone who thinks before, what he wants to cook buys more targeted and provides more variety. Generally good: Buy fresh and seasonal goods as much as possible. It tastes better and is often cheaper.

**FRUIT AND VEGETABLES**

Season: Buy seasonally. Tomatoes, radishes or strawberries have a long journey in the winter and come mostly from the greenhouse. This is at the expense of taste and vitamin content.

Fresh or frozen: Let withered spinach or yellowish broccoli lie down. When in doubt, frozen vegetables are better. It is processed harvest fresh, the vitamin content is higher and the taste better than long-stored goods. Sometimes the handle to preserve is worthwhile. Example tomatoes: Here come fully ripe fruit in the can.

Mature or immature: Ripe fruits give on finger pressure usually slightly and smell good. Some fruits and vegetables can also be bought immature. Apples, bananas, kiwis or avocados ripen at home.

Appearance: The appearance is often secondary: the shinier the apple, the more likely it has been treated with pesticides. You should also ignore size and commercial classes: Especially small fruits are often big in taste.

Packaged fruit: Should you weigh. For cardboard trays, check that the soil is moist. Then down is slush.

Street stalls. Small greengrocers often offer particularly appetizing greens. But you should intensively brush it at home. Car exhaust and abraded brake pads are deposited.

FISH

Storage: If possible, fresh fish should be on ice and covered with it. Also packaged smoked fish must be sufficiently cooled. As a precaution, do not buy goods that have almost reached the end of their shelf life.

Appearance and smell: Moist, bright red gills, shiny skin, clear mucus and clear eyes characterize fresh fish. If the fish smells severe, do without it.

Fish sticks: Are a viable alternative for anyone who likes neither the sight nor the taste of raw fish. They contain all essential Ingredients. But: A stick is 35 percent breadcrumbs, which fat and energy levels grow enormously. Who wants to reduce the fat content, can bake the fish fingers in the oven.

Shellfish: Filtering with food also pollutants from the water. If possible, avoid mussels from near-industrial regions. Mussel meat spoils even easier than fish. Open mussels have to close on pressure themselves. Otherwise they should be sorted out.

Surimi: Is not an exquisite delicacy, but a crustacean or crabmeat from fish leftovers. It can also contain dyes and is flavored with sugar, salt and spices. Allergy sufferers should carefully examine the list of Ingredients.

Sustainable fishing: The oceans are overfished. About half of the food fish comes from farms today (aquaculture). If you have wild fish, pay attention to the MSC seal or else opt for organic aquaculture.

**MEAT**

Appearance: Good meat should not be absolutely lean. A light marbling not only serves better cooking, but also the taste. Fresh meat should not be too light, too shiny, dry or too moist.

Self-service: Take a good look at meat: the blood on the bone must be fresh and bright red.

Cool. Meat spoils quickly at room temperature. That means go home quickly and put it in the refrigerator or prepare it.

Whitewashing: Sometimes the rosy fresh offer from the meat counter on the way home gets a pale, unappealing color. This may be due to the lighting in the counter. Anyone who believes that they have been "duped" should change the butcher.

## CHEESE

Arrangement: Cheese should be arranged by kinship, ie hard and white and white mold with white cheese. Molds can migrate, and taste notes can influence them.

Aroma: Buy cheese in one piece. Pre-cut, it dries out and quickly loses its aroma. Press soft cheese lightly. Young cheese is firm, more mature gives way

# Chapter 6

# Breakfast Meal Plan

## *Blueberry Scones*

Preparation time: 10 minutes

Cooking time: 15 minutes

Servings: 12

**Ingredients:**

Baking powder -2 tsp.

Vanilla -2 tsp.

Stevia -.5 c.

Raspberries -.75 c.

Almond flour -1.5 c.

Beaten eggs -3

**Directions:**

Allow the oven to heat up to 375 degrees and add some parchment paper to a baking sheet.

Take out a bowl and beat together the almond flour, eggs, baking powder, vanilla, and stevia. Fold the raspberries in.

Scoop this batter onto the baking sheet. Add to the oven. After 15 minutes, take the scones out and let them cool down before serving.

**Nutrition Value:**

Calories: 133

Fats: 8g

Carbs: 4g

Protein: 2g

## *Cinnamon Porridge*

Preparation time: 5 minutes

Cooking time: 5 minutes

Servings: 4

**Ingredients:**

Cinnamon -1 tsp.

Stevia -1.5 tsp.

Butter -1 Tbsp.

Flaxseed meal -2 Tbsp.

Oat bran -2 Tbsp.

Shredded coconut -.5 c.

Heavy cream -1 c.

Water -2 c.

**Directions:**

Combine all of your Ingredients into a pot and mix around.

Place it on a low flame and bring to a boil. Stir it well when it is boiling and then remove from the heat.

Divide into four servings and set aside for a bit to thicken.

**Nutrition Value:**

Calories: 171

Fats: 16g

Carbs: 6g

Protein: 2g

## *Scotch Eggs*

Preparation time: 15 minutes

Cooking time: 25 minutes

Servings: 6

Ingredients:

Pepper -.5 tsp.

Salt -.33 tp.

Garlic powder -1.5 tsp.

Breakfast sausage -1.5 c.

Peeled hard-boiled eggs

## Directions:

Allow the oven to heat up to 400 degrees. Add the sausage to a bowl and add the garlic, pepper, and salt.

Divide this into 6 equal parts and add to some baking paper. Flatten them out and then place the hard boiled eggs on top. Wrap the sausage around the egg.

Arrange onto a baking sheet and place into the oven. After 25 minutes, take these out and allow to cool down.

## Nutrition Value:

Calories: 258

Fats: 21g

Carbs: 1g

Protein: 17g

## *Breakfast Tacos*

Preparation time: 10 minutes

Cooking time: 5 minutes

Servings: 2

## Ingredients:

Pepper

Salt

Tabasco sauce

Cilantro sprigs -4

Butter -1 Tbsp.

Sliced avocado -.5

Eggs -4

Low carb tortillas -2

**Directions:**

Whisk the eggs until they are smooth. Take out a skillet and heat up the butter on it.

Add the prepared eggs and spread it out. cook until done and then move to a bowl. Warm up the tortillas and then put on a platter.

Spread mayo over one side of the tortillas. Divide up the egg on the tortilla and top with the avocado and cilantro. Add the pepper, salt, and pepper sauce.

Roll up the tortillas and then serve or store.

**Nutrition Value:**

Calories: 289

Fats: 27g

Carbs: 6g

Protein: 7g

# *Vanilla Smoothie*

Preparation time: 2 minutes

Cooking time: 0

Servings: 1

**Ingredients:**

Whipped cream

Liquid stevia -3 drops

Vanilla -.5 tsp.

Ice cubes -4

Water -.25 c.

Mascarpone cheese -.5 c.

Egg yolks -2

**Directions:**

Take out your blender and add in all the Ingredients.

Place the lid on top and blend. When the Ingredients are well mixed, pour into a glass and serve.

**Nutrition Value:**

Calories: 650

Fats: 64g

Carbs: 4g

Protein: 12g

## *Blackberry Egg Bake*

Preparation time:  10 minutes

Cooking time: 15 minutes

Servings: 4

**Ingredients:**

Chopped rosemary -1 tsp.

Orange zest -.5 tsp.

Salt

Vanilla -.25 tsp.

Grated ginger -1 tsp.

Coconut flour -3 Tbsp.

Butter -1 Tbsp.

Egg -5

Blackberries -.5 c.

**Directions:**

Allow the oven to heat up to 350 degrees. Take out a blender and add all the Ingredients inside to blend well.

Pour this into each muffin cup and then add the blackberries on top. Place into the oven to bake.

After 15 minutes, take the dish out and store!

**Nutrition Value:**

Calories: 144

Fats: 10g

Carbs: 2g

Protein: 8.5g

## *Coconut Pancakes*

Preparation time: 10 minutes

Cooking time: 5 minutes

Servings: 2

**Ingredients:**

Maple syrup -4 Tbsp.

Shredded coconut -.25 c.

Salt

Erythritol -.5 Tbsp.

Cinnamon -1 tsp.

Almond flour -1 Tbsp.

Cream cheese -2 oz.

Eggs -2

**Directions:**

Beat the eggs together before adding in the almond flour and cream cheese.

Now add in the rest of the Ingredients and stir until well combined.

Take out a frying pan and fry the pancakes on both sides. Add to a plate and sprinkle some coconut on top.

**Nutrition Value:**

Calories: 575

Fats: 51g

Carbs: 3.5g

Protein: 19g

## *Chocolate Chip Waffles*

Preparation time: 8 minutes

Cooking time: 10 minutes

Servings: 2

**Ingredients:**

Maple syrup -.5 c.

Cacao nibs -50g

Salt

Butter -2 Tbsp.

Separated eggs -2

Protein powder -2 scoops

**Directions:**

Take out a bowl and beat the egg whites until soft peaks form. In a second bowl mix the butter, protein powder, and egg yolks.

Now fold the egg whites into this mixture and add the cacao nibs and salt.

Pour the mixture into a waffle maker and let it cook until golden brown on both sides. Serve with maple syrup.

**Nutrition Value:**

Calories: 400

Fats: 26g

Carbs: 4.5g

Protein: 34g

## *Chocolate And Peanut Butter Muffins*

Preparation time: 20 minutes

Cooking time: 20 minutes

Servings: 6

**Ingredients:**

Eggs -2

Almond milk -.33 c.

Peanut butter -.33 c.

Salt

Baking powder -1 tsp.

Erythritol -.5 c.

Almond flour -1 c.

**Directions:**

Bring out a bowl and mix the salt, baking powder, erythritol, and almond flour together. Add the eggs, almond milk, and peanut butter next.

Finally, mix in the cacao nibs before pouring this into a muffin tin.

Allow the oven to heat up to 350 degrees. Place the muffin tray into the oven to bake.

After 25 minutes, the muffins are done and you can store.


**Nutrition Value:**

Calories: 265

Fats: 20.5g

Carbs: 2g

Protein: 7.5g

## *Blender Pancakes*

Preparation time: 5 minutes:

Cooking time: 5 minutes

Servings: 1

**Ingredients:**

Salt

Cinnamon

Protein powder -1 scoop

Eggs -2

Cream cheese -2 oz.

**Directions:**

Add the salt, cinnamon, protein powder, eggs, and cream cheese to a blender and combine well.

Take out a skillet and fry the batter on both sides until done. Serve warm.

**Nutrition Value:**

Calories: 450

Fat: 29g

Carbs: 4g

Protein: 41g

# *Butter Coffee*

Preparation time: 5 minutes

Cooking time

Servings: 1

**Ingredients:**

Coconut oil -1 Tbsp.

Butter -1 Tbsp.

Coffee -2 Tbsp.

Water -1 c.

**Directions:**

Bring out a pan and boil the water inside. When the water is boiling, add in the coffee, coconut oil, and butter.

Once these are all melted and hot, pour into a cup through a strainer and enjoy.

**Nutrition Value:**

Calories: 230

Fat: 25g

Carbs: 0g

Protein: 0g

# *Mocha Chia Pudding*

Preparation time: 5 minutes

Cooking time: 10 minutes

Servings: 2

Ingredients:

Cacao nibs -2 Tbsp.

Swerve -1 Tbsp.

Vanilla -1 Tbsp.

Coconut cream -.33 g

Chia seeds -55g

Water -2 c.

Herbal coffee -2 Tbsp.

**Directions:**

Brew the herbal coffee with some hot water until the liquid is reduced in half. Strain the coffee before mixing in with the vanilla, swerve, and coconut cream.

Add in the chia seeds and cacao nibs net. Pour into some cups and place in the fridge for 30 minutes before serving.

**Nutrition Value:**

Calories: 257

Fat: 20.25g

Carbs: 2.25g

Protein: 7g

## *Keto Green Eggs*

Preparation time: 5 minutes

Cooking time: 12 minutes

Servings:2

**Ingredients:**

Ground cayenne -.25 tsp.

Ground cumin -.25 tsp.

Eggs -4

Chopped parsley -.5 c.

Chopped cilantro -.5 c.

Thyme leaves -1 tsp.

Garlic cloves -2

Coconut oil -1 Tbsp.

Butter -2 Tbsp.

**Directions:**

Melt the butter and coconut oil in a skillet before adding the garlic and frying. Add in the thyme, parsley and cilantro and cook another 3 minutes.

At this time, add in the eggs and season. Cover with a lid and let this cook for another 5 minutes before serving.

**Nutrition Value:**

Calories: 311

Fat: 27.5g

Carbs: 4g

Protein: 12.8g

## *Cheddar Souffles*

Preparation time: 15 minutes

Cooking time: 25 minutes

Servings: 8

**Ingredients:**

Cheddar cheese -2 c.

Heavy cream -.75 c.

Cayenne pepper -.25 tsp.

Xanthan gum -.5 tsp.

Pepper -.5 tsp.

Ground mustard -1 tsp.

Salt -1 tsp.

Almond flour -.5 c.

Salt -1 pinch

Cream of tartar -.25 tsp.

Eggs -6

Chopped chives -.25 c.

**Directions:**

Allow the oven to heat up to 350 degrees. Take out a bowl and mix all the Ingredients besides the eggs and cream of tartar together.

Separate the egg whites and yolks and add the yolks in with the first mixture. Beat the egg whites and cream of tartar until you get stiff peaks to form.

Take this mixture and add into the other mixture. When done, pour into the ramekins and place in the oven.

After 25 minutes, these are done and you can serve or store.

**Nutrition Value:**

Calories: 288

Fat: 21g

Carbs: 3g

Protein: 14g

# *Ricotta Pie*

Preparation time: 10 minutes

Cooking time: 30 minutes

Servings: 6

**Ingredients:**

Mozzarella -1 c.

Eggs -3

Ricotta cheese -2 c.

Swiss chard -8 c.

Garlic clove -1

Chopped onion -.5 c.

Olive oil -1 Tbsp.

Mild sausage -1 lb.

Pepper

Salt

Nutmeg

Parmesan -.25 c.

**Directions:**

Heat up the garlic, onion, and oil on a pan. When those are warm, add in the swiss chard and fry to make the leaves wilt.

Add in the nutmeg and set it aside. In a new bowl, beat the eggs before adding in the cheeses. Now add in the prepared swiss chard mixture.

Roll out the sausage and press it into a pie tart. Pour the filing inside. Allow the oven to heat to 350 degrees.

Place the pie inside and let it bake. After 30 minutes, it is done and you can store or serve.

**Nutrition Value:**

Calories: 344

Fat: 27g

Carbs: 4g

Protein: 23g

## *Vegetarian Red Coconut Curry*

Servings: 2

Preparation time: 35 mins

**Ingredients**

¾ cup spinach

¼ medium onion, chopped

1 teaspoon ginger, minced

1 cup broccoli florets

4 tablespoons coconut oil

1 teaspoon garlic, minced

2 teaspoons coconut aminos

1 tablespoon red curry paste

2 teaspoons soy sauce

½ cup coconut cream

**Directions**

Heat 2 tablespoons of coconut oil in a pan and add garlic and onions.

Sauté for about 3 minutes and add broccoli.

Sauté for about 3 minutes and move vegetables to the side of the pan.

Add curry paste and cook for about 1 minute.

Mix well and add spinach, cooking for about 3 minutes.

Add coconut cream, remaining coconut oil, ginger, soy sauce and coconut aminos.

Allow it to simmer for about 10 minutes and dish out to serve.

**Nutrition Value:**

Calories: 439  Carbs: 12g  Fats: 44g  Proteins: 3.6g  Sodium: 728mg
Sugar: 3.5g

## *Zucchini Noodles With Avocado Sauce*

Servings: 2

Preparation time: 10 mins

**Ingredients**

1¼ cup basil

4 tablespoons pine nuts

1 zucchini, spiralized

1/3 cup water

2 tablespoons lemon juice

2 cherry tomatoes, sliced

1 avocado

**Directions**

Put all the Ingredients except the cherry tomatoes and zucchini in a blender and blend until smooth.

Mix together the blended sauce and zucchini noodles and cherry tomatoes in a serving bowl and serve.

**Nutrition Value:**

Calories: 366   Carbs: 19.7g   Fats: 32g   Proteins: 7.1g   Sodium: 27mg   Sugar: 6.4g

## *Tomato Basil And Mozzarella Galette*

Servings: 2

Preparation time: 35 mins

**Ingredients**

1 large egg

1 teaspoon garlic powder

¾ cup almond flour

2 tablespoons mozzarella liquid

¼ cup Parmesan cheese, shredded

3 leaves fresh basil

2 plum tomatoes

1½ tablespoons pesto

1/3-ounce Mozzarella cheese

**Directions**

Preheat oven to 365 degrees F and line a cookie sheet with parchment paper.

Mix together the garlic powder, almond flour and mozzarella liquid in a bowl.

Add Parmesan cheese and egg and mix to form a dough.

Form balls out of this dough mixture and transfer on the cookie sheet.

Press the dough balls with a fork and spread pesto over the centre of the crust evenly.

Layer mozzarella, tomatoes and basil leaves, and fold the edges of the crust up and over the filling.

Transfer in the oven and bake for about 20 minutes.

Dish out to serve.

**Nutrition Value:**

Calories: 396  Carbs: 17.6g  Fats: 29.2g  Proteins: 17.5g  Sodium: 199mg  Sugar: 6.2g

## *Cheesy Spaghetti Squash With Pesto*

Servings: 2

Preparation time: 25 mins

**Ingredients**

½ tablespoon olive oil

¼ cup whole milk ricotta cheese

1/8 cup basil pesto

1 cup cooked spaghetti squash, drained

Salt and black pepper, to taste

2 oz fresh mozzarella cheese, cubed

**Directions**

Preheat the oven to 375 degrees F and grease a casserole dish.

Mix together squash and olive oil in a medium-sized bowl and season with salt and black pepper.

Put the squash in the casserole dish and top with ricotta and mozzarella cheese.

Bake for about 10 minutes and remove from the oven.

Drizzle the pesto over the top and serve hot.

**Nutrition Value:**

Calories: 169   Carbs: 6.2g   Fats: 11.3g   Proteins: 11.9g   Sodium: 217mg  Sugar: 0.1g

## *Vegan Sesame Tofu And Eggplant*

Servings: 2

Preparation time: 30 mins

**Ingredients**

½ cup cilantro, chopped

2 tablespoons toasted sesame oil

½ teaspoon crushed red pepper flakes

Mix together all the Ingredients in a bowl and stir until well combined.

Refrigerate for about 3 hours and serve chilled.

Put the salad into a container for meal prepping and refrigerate for about 2 days.

**Nutrition Value:**

Calories: 336  Carbohydrates: 2g  Protein: 27.2g  Fat: 25.2g  Sugar: 1.2g  Sodium: 926mg

## *Beef Sausage Pancakes*

Servings: 2

Preparation time: 30 mins

**Ingredients**

4 gluten-free Italian beef sausages, sliced

1 tablespoon olive oil

1/3 large red bell peppers, seeded and sliced thinly

1/3 cup spinach

¾ teaspoon garlic powder

1/3 large green bell peppers, seeded and sliced thinly

¾ cup heavy whipped cream

Salt and black pepper, to taste

½ eggplant, julienned

½ pound block firm tofu, pressed

1½ tablespoons rice vinegar

1 clove garlic, finely minced

1 teaspoon Swerve

½ tablespoon olive oil

1/8 cup sesame seeds

Salt and black pepper, to taste

1/8 cup soy sauce

**Directions**

Preheat the oven to 200 degrees F.

Mix together cilantro, eggplant, rice vinegar, half of toasted sesame oil, garlic, red pepper flakes and Swerve in a bowl.

Heat olive oil in a skillet and add the marinated eggplant.

Sauté for about 4 minutes and transfer the eggplant noodles to an oven safe dish.

Cover with a foil and place into the oven to keep warm.

Spread the sesame seeds on a plate and press both sides of each piece of tofu into the seeds.

Add remaining sesame oil and tofu to the skillet and fry for about 5 minutes.

Pour soy sauce into the pan and cook until the tofu slices are browned.

Remove the eggplant noodles from the oven and top with tofu to serve.

**Nutrition Value:**

Calories: 333  Carbs: 13.9g  Fats: 26.6g  Proteins: 13.3g  Sodium: 918mg  Sugar: 4.5g

## *Cheesy Spinach Puffs*

Servings: 2

Preparation time: 25 mins

**Ingredients**

½ cup almond flour

1 large egg

¼ cup feta cheese, crumbled

½ teaspoon kosher salt

½ teaspoon garlic powder

1½ tablespoons heavy whipping cream

**Directions**

Preheat the oven to 350 degrees F and grease a cookie sheet.

Put all the Ingredients in a blender and pulse until smooth.

Allow to cool down and form 1-inch balls from this mixture.

Arrange on a cookie sheet and transfer into the oven.

Bake for about 12 minutes and dish out to serve.

**Nutrition Value:**

Calories: 294   Carbs: 7.8g   Fats: 24g   Proteins: 12.2g   Sodium: 840mg  Sugar: 1.1g

## *Lobster Salad*

Servings: 2

Preparation time: 15 mins

**Ingredients**

¼ yellow onion, chopped

¼ yellow bell pepper, seeded and chopped

¾ pound cooked lobster meat, shredded

1 celery stalk, chopped

Black pepper, to taste

¼ cup avocado mayonnaise

**Directions**

## Directions

Mix together all the Ingredients in a bowl except whipped cream and keep aside.

Put butter and half of the mixture in a skillet and cook for about 6 minutes on both sides.

Repeat with the remaining mixture and dish out.

Beat whipped cream in another bowl until smooth.

Serve the beef sausage pancakes with whipped cream.

For meal prepping, it is compulsory to gently slice the sausages before mixing with other Ingredients.

## Nutrition Value:

Calories: 415  Carbohydrates: 7g  Protein: 29.5g  Fat: 31.6g  Sugar: 4.3g  Sodium: 1040mg

## *Holiday Chicken Salad*

Servings: 2

Preparation time: 25 mins

## Ingredients

1 celery stalk, chopped

1½ cups cooked grass-fed chicken, chopped

¼ cup fresh cranberries

¼ cup sour cream

½ apple, chopped

¼ yellow onion, chopped

1/8 cup almonds, toasted and chopped

2-ounce feta cheese, crumbled

¼ cup avocado mayonnaise

Salt and black pepper, to taste

**Directions**

Stir together all the Ingredients in a bowl except almonds and cheese.

Top with almonds and cheese to serve.

Meal Prep Tip: Don't add almonds and cheese in the salad if you want to store the salad. Cover with a plastic wrap and refrigerate to serve.

**Nutrition Value:**

Calories: 336   Carbohydrates: 8.8g   Protein: 24.5g   Fat: 23.2g Sugar: 5.4g  Sodium: 383mg

## *Luncheon Fancy Salad*

Servings: 2

Preparation time: 40 mins

## Ingredients

6-ounce cooked salmon, chopped

1 tablespoon fresh dill, chopped

Salt and black pepper, to taste

4 hard-boiled grass-fed eggs, peeled and cubed

2 celery stalks, chopped

½ yellow onion, chopped

¾ cup avocado mayonnaise

## Directions

Put all the Ingredients in a bowl and mix until well combined.

Cover with a plastic wrap and refrigerate for about 3 hours to serve.

For meal prepping, put the salad in a container and refrigerate for up to 3 days.

## Nutrition Value:

Calories: 303  Carbohydrates: 1.7g  Protein: 10.3g  Fat: 30g  Sugar: 1g  Sodium: 314mg

## *Italian Platter*

Servings: 2

Preparation time: 45 mins

## Ingredients

1 garlic clove, minced

5-ounce fresh button mushrooms, sliced

1/8 cup unsalted butter

¼ teaspoon dried thyme

1/3 cup heavy whipping cream

Salt and black pepper, to taste

2 -6-ounce grass-fed New York strip steaks

**Directions**

Preheat the grill to medium heat and grease it.

Season the steaks with salt and black pepper, and transfer to the grill.

Grill steaks for about 10 minutes on each side and dish out in a platter.

Put butter, mushrooms, salt and black pepper in a pan and cook for about 10 minutes.

Add thyme and garlic and thyme and sauté for about 1 minute.

Stir in the cream and let it simmer for about 5 minutes.

Top the steaks with mushroom sauce and serve hot immediately.

Meal Prep Tip: You can store the mushroom sauce in refrigerator for about 2 days. Season the steaks carefully with salt and black pepper to avoid low or high quantities.

**Nutrition Value:**

Calories: 332    Carbohydrates: 3.2g    Protein: 41.8g    Fat: 20.5g
Sugar: 1.3g  Sodium: 181mg

# *Meat Loaf*

Servings: 12

Preparation time: 1 hour 15 mins

## Ingredients

1 garlic clove, minced

½ teaspoon dried thyme, crushed

½ pound grass-fed lean ground beef

1 organic egg, beaten

Salt and black pepper, to taste

¼ cup onions, chopped

1/8 cup sugar-free ketchup

2 cups mozzarella cheese, freshly grated

¼ cup green bell pepper, seeded and chopped

½ cup cheddar cheese, grated

1 cup fresh spinach, chopped

## Directions

Preheat the oven to 350 degrees F and grease a baking dish.

Put all the Ingredients in a bowl except spinach and cheese and mix well.

Arrange the meat over a wax paper and top with spinach and cheese.

Roll the paper around the mixture to form a meatloaf.

Remove the wax paper and transfer the meat loaf in the baking dish.

Put it in the oven and bake for about 1 hour.

Dish out and serve hot.

Meal Prep Tip: Let the meat loafs cool for about 10 minutes to bring them to room temperature before serving.

**Nutrition Value:**

Calories: 439  Carbohydrates: 8g  Protein: 40.8g  Fat: 26g  Sugar: 1.6g  Sodium: 587mg

## *Grilled Steak*

Servings: 2

Preparation time: 15 mins

**Ingredients**

¼ cup unsalted butter

2 garlic cloves, minced

¾ pound beef top sirloin steaks

¾ teaspoon dried rosemary, crushed

2 oz. parmesan cheese, shredded

Salt and black pepper, to taste

**Directions**

Preheat the grill and grease it.

Season the sirloin steaks with salt and black pepper.

Transfer the steaks on the grill and cook for about 5 minutes on each side.

Dish out the steaks in plates and keep aside.

Meanwhile, put butter and garlic in a pan and heat until melted.

Pour it on the steaks and serve hot.

Divide the steaks in 2 containers and refrigerate for about 3 days for meal prepping purpose. Reheat in microwave before serving.

**Nutrition Value:**

Calories: 383   Carbohydrates: 1.5g    Protein: 41.4g   Fat: 23.6g
Sugar: 0g  Sodium: 352mg

# Chapter 7

# Lunch Meal Plan

### *Roasted Veggie Salad*

**Total time:** 30 minutes

**Ingredients**

2 cups cubed butternut squash (I keep the skin on but you can remove it if you wish)

2 cups cubed sweet potato

2 carrots, chopped into chunks

2 large Portobello mushrooms, thickly sliced

2 large zucchinis, cut into chunks

1 head of broccoli, cut into florets

2 tbsp. sunflower seeds

2 tbsp. pumpkin seeds

3 tbsp. olive oil (I've added the oil in here because it's quite a lot and it adjusts the calorie count)

Salt and pepper, to taste

### Directions

Preheat the oven to 356 degrees Fahrenheit and prepare a tray by lining it with baking paper.

Place all Ingredients onto the tray and add a sprinkle of salt and pepper.

Combine the Ingredients together with your hands, making sure everything gets coated in olive oil.

Place into the oven and bake for approximately 30 minutes or until the veggies are soft and the seeds are toasted.

Divide into your 4 containers, cover and place into the fridge until needed.

## *Pita Pockets With Lamb And Salad*

**Total time:** 20 minutes

### Ingredients

12 oz. lamb steaks, cut into cubes

1 tsp. ground cumin

Salt and pepper, to taste

4 whole-meal pita breads

2 cups salad greens (mixed kale, lettuce and arugula is ideal)

4 tbsp. plain yogurt

1 lemon, cut into quarters

**Directions**

Drizzle some olive oil into a fry pan and place over a medium heat.

Add the lamb, cumin, salt and pepper and stir to combine, sauté for about 7 minutes or until the lamb cubes are cooked but still a little pink.

Make a slit in each pita bread and fill each one with mixed salad greens, lamb, and a drizzle of yogurt.

Place the filled pitas into your 4 containers and place a lemon quarter in each one so you can squeeze it over the pita when you're ready to eat!

Cover the containers and store in the fridge until needed.

## *Sticky Chicken And Broccoli Prep Bowls*

**Total time:** 30 minutes

**Ingredients**

2 tbsp. honey

2 tsp. soy sauce (tamari is best)

4 boneless, skinless chicken thighs

1 head of broccoli, cut into florets

1 tsp. sesame oil

**Directions**

Drizzle some olive oil into a frying pan and place over a medium heat.

Add the honey and soy sauce, place the chicken thighs into the pan and stir to coat in soy and honey, sauté for approximately 15 minutes or until the chicken is almost cooked.

Add the broccoli to the pan, increase the heat to high, splash a few teaspoons of water into the pan and immediate place a lid onto the pan – this will steam the broccoli.

Once the water has evaporated, remove the lid and check that the chicken has cooked through and the broccoli is cooked yet crunchy.

Drizzle the sesame oil over the broccoli before dividing the chicken and broccoli between your 4 containers.

Cover and store in the fridge until needed!

## *Quinoa And Fresh Greens Salad*

**Total time:** 25 minutes

**Ingredients**

1 cup dry quinoa

1 ½ cups (12floz) salt-reduced chicken broth/stock

3 cups shredded lettuce (use any, I use iceberg)

2 cups baby spinach leaves

2 green bell peppers, core and seeds removed, sliced

3 oz. feta cheese, cut into small chunks

Salt and pepper, to taste

**Directions**

Thoroughly rinse the quinoa in a sieve to remove the bitter outer layer.

Bring the chicken broth to the boil in a small pot and add the quinoa, stir to combine then turn the heat down to a simmer, cover, and cook for 12-15 minutes or until the liquid has disappeared and the quinoa is soft.

Divide the cooked quinoa between your 4 containers, then divide the lettuce, spinach, bell peppers and feta between the containers and place on top of the quinoa.

Sprinkle with salt and pepper and a drizzle of olive oil to finish.

Cover and place into the fridge until needed!

## *Homemade Hummus, Tomato, And Ham Rice Wafer Stacks*

**Total time:** 20 minutes

**Ingredients**

1 can of chickpeas, drained

1 tbsp. tahini

1 garlic clove

4 tbsp. olive oil

1 lemon

Salt and pepper, to taste

12 rice wafers

2 large tomatoes, sliced

4 large slices of deli ham

**Directions**

Make the hummus by placing the chickpeas, tahini, garlic clove, olive oil, juice of one lemon, salt and pepper into a blender or food processor and blending until smooth.

Wrap your rice wafers in plastic wrap to keep them fresh and place them into the pantry.

Place a good drop of hummus into one corner of your airtight containers, then divide the tomato and ham between the containers too.

Place the lid onto your containers and place them into the fridge until needed.

When it's time to pack your lunch into your work bag, simply place a container of toppings into your bag and grab a packet of wrapped rice wafers too.

Assemble just before eating for a fresh and crunchy lunch!

## *Grilled Salmon And Seasonal Greens*

**Total time:** 30 minutes

**Ingredients**

4 small-medium salmon filets

Salt and pepper, to taste

Olive oil

1 head of broccoli, cut into florets

2 large zucchinis, chopped into chunks

1 tsp. sesame oil

**Directions**

Preheat the oven to 356 degrees Fahrenheit and line a baking tray with baking paper, place the salmon filets onto the tray and sprinkle with salt, pepper and a little olive oil.

Place into the oven and bake for approximately 12 minutes or until cooked to your liking.

As the salmon cooks, prepare the greens by placing a pot of water over a high heat and bringing to the boil, place a steaming basket or double boiler over the pot and place the greens inside, place the lid onto the basket.

Steam the veggies for a few minutes until just cooked, sprinkle with the sesame oil and some salt and pepper.

Place a salmon filet into each container and divide the veggies between each container.

Place the lid onto each container and place into the fridge to store before serving.

Eat hot or cold!

## *Chicken, Strawberry, And Black Rice Salad*

**Total time:** 40 minutes

**Ingredients**

2 cups dry black rice

1 large chicken breast

Olive oil

Salt and pepper, to taste

1 cup strawberries, stalks removed, sliced

1 lemon

**Directions**

Preheat the oven to 356 degrees Fahrenheit and line a baking tray with baking paper.

Place the rice into a pot and add 4 cups of water and a pinch of salt, bring to the boil then reduce to a simmer, cover and let simmer until the water has disappeared and the rice is cooked.

While the rice is cooking, cook the chicken by placing it onto the lined baking tray, drizzling with olive oil, and sprinkling with salt and pepper, bake in the preheated oven for approximately 20 minutes or until cooked through.

Shred the cooked chicken breast and add to the pot with the cooked black rice.

Place the strawberries into the pot and squeeze in the juice of one lemon.

Season with salt and pepper before stirring to combine.

Divide between your 4 containers, cover and store in the fridge until needed!

## *Cauliflower Rice And Chili Chicken*

**Total time:** 30 minutes

**Ingredients**

1 head of cauliflower, core removed, florets cut into chunks

Salt and pepper, to taste

4 boneless, skinless chicken thighs

2 tbsp. olive oil

1 fresh red chili, finely chopped

1 garlic clove, crushed

1 lemon, cut into quarters

**Directions**

Preheat the oven to 356 degrees Fahrenheit and line a baking tray with baking paper.

Place the cauliflower into a food processor and blend until it resembles the size and consistency of rice.

Place the cauliflower into a bowl and sprinkle with salt and pepper, place in the microwave and cook on HIGH for 1 minute increments until cooked through.

Place the chicken thighs onto the lined baking tray and sprinkle the olive oil, chili, garlic, salt and pepper on top rub to combine and make sure the chicken is well-coated.

Place the chicken into the preheated oven and bake for approximately 20 minutes or until the chicken is cooked through.

Divide the cauliflower rice between the 4 containers and place a chicken thigh into each container on top of the "rice".

Place a lemon quarter into each container, cover and place into the fridge until needed!

## *Loaded Broccoli Salad With Toasted Seeds*

**Total time:** 20 minutes

**Ingredients**

Olive oil

1 large head of broccoli, stalk removed, cut into florets

¼ red onion, finely chopped

2 tbsp. pumpkin seeds

2 tbsp. sunflower seeds

3 tbsp. grated Parmesan cheese

Salt and pepper, to taste

**Directions**

Drizzle some olive oil into a frying pan and place over a medium heat.

Add the broccoli and sauté for a few minutes.

Pour a few tablespoons of water into the pan and immediately place a lid on top to trap the steam, this will steam the broccoli.

Once the water has evaporated and the broccoli is cooked but still has a "bite", add the red onion, pumpkin seeds and sunflower seeds, continue cooking for about 1 minute until the seeds are gently toasted.

Divide the broccoli mixture between your 4 containers and sprinkle the Parmesan over each one.

Finish with a sprinkle of salt and pepper and a little drizzle of olive oil.

Cover and place into the fridge until needed!

## *White Bean And Tomato Salad With Balsamic Dressing*

**Total time:** 10 minutes

**Ingredients**

2 cans white beans, drained

3 ripe tomatoes, cut into chunks

Small handful of fresh basil, roughly chopped

2 tbsp. balsamic vinegar mixed with 2 tablespoons of olive oil

Salt and pepper, to taste

**Directions**

Place the beans, tomatoes, basil, balsamic, olive oil, salt and pepper into a small bowl and mix to combine.

Divide into your 4 containers, cover and place into the fridge to store until needed.

Eat cold!

## *One-Tray Chicken Thigh And Root Veggie Baked "Bowls"*

**Total time:** 35 minutes

**Ingredients**

4 boneless, skinless chicken thighs

2 carrots, cut into small chunks

2 parsnips, peeled and cut into chunks

2 raw beets, cut into chunks

1 large red onion, cut into wedges

1 tsp. mixed dried herbs

Olive oil

Salt and pepper, to taste

1 lemon, cut into quarters

**Directions**

Preheat the oven to 356 degrees Fahrenheit and line a baking tray with baking paper.

Place the chicken thighs, carrots, parsnips, beets, onion, herbs and a drizzle of olive oil onto the tray, add a pinch of salt and pepper and combine all of the Ingredients with your hands.

Place the tray into the oven and bake for approximately 30 minutes or until the chicken is cooked through and the veggies are soft.

Divide the chicken and veggies between the 4 containers and place a lemon quarter into each container.

Place into the fridge to store until needed!

## Cold Soba Noodle Salad With Cashews, Carrot And Tofu

**Total time:** 20 minutes

**Ingredients**

14 oz. dry soba noodles

2 tbsp. sesame oil

2 tbsp. soy sauce

1 tbsp. honey

9 oz. firm tofu, sliced

1/3 cup raw cashew nuts

2 carrots, peeled and chopped into small pieces

**Directions**

Place a pot of water over a high heat, bring to the boil and add the soba noodles, cook until soft.

While the noodles are cooking, drizzle the sesame oil, soy sauce and honey into a small non-stick fry pan and place over a medium heat.

Place the tofu slices into the hot pan and cook for a couple of minutes on each side until golden.

Drain the noodles and place into a bowl.

Add the cashews, carrots, and cooked tofu with any oil/soy sauce left over in the fry pan.

Stir to combine.

Divide into your 4 containers, cover and place into the fridge to store until needed!

Best eaten cold!

## *Basil, Tomato And Haloumi Salad With Cos And Cucumber*

**Total time:** 20 minutes

**Ingredients**

7 oz. halloumi cheese, sliced into 12 slices

2 cos or Romaine lettuces, roughly chopped

1 cup chopped cucumber

3 large tomatoes, sliced

Large handful of fresh basil, roughly chopped

2 tbsp. apple cider vinegar mixed with 2 tbsp. olive oil

**Directions**

Heat a non-stick frying pan over a high heat.

Add the halloumi slices to the pan and cook on both sides until golden.

Divide the lettuce, cucumber, tomatoes, basil, and halloumi between the 4 containers.

Sprinkle with salt and pepper and the oil/vinegar mixture, gently toss to combine and coat with dressing.

Cover and place into the fridge to store until needed.

## *Prepped Topping Packs For Rice Wafers*

**Total time:** 10 minutes

**Ingredients**

1 cup cottage cheese

4 tbsp. chopped chives

1 fresh tomato, sliced

4 slices of deli ham or turkey

4 tbsp. peanut butter

1 banana, cut into 4 chunks

(plus 4 rice wafers per lunch serving)

**Directions**

Place the cottage cheese, chives, tomato, ham or turkey, peanut butter, and banana into a container with separated compartments.

Cover and place into the fridge to store until needed.

Wrap the rice wafers in sealable bags or plastic wrap, or keep them in an airtight container at work to pull out whenever you need them!

## *Minced Lamb Meat Balls With Yogurt And Cucumber Dip*

**Total time:** 25 minutes

**Ingredients:**

17.5 oz. minced lamb

½ red onion, finely chopped

1 egg

½ cup almond flour

Salt and pepper, to taste

Olive oil

½ cup plain Greek yogurt

¾ cup finely chopped cucumber

**Directions**

Place the minced lamb, red onion, egg, almond flour, salt and pepper into a bowl and stir to combine.

Drizzle some olive oil into a non-stick fry pan and place over a medium heat.

Roll the lamb mixture into 16 balls and place them in 2 batches into the hot pan, cook for about 7 minutes, turning a few times until golden and cooked through.

Stir together the yogurt and cucumber in a small bowl.

Place 4 lamb balls into each container and place a drop of yogurt mixture over top.

Cover and place into the fridge to store until needed.

Eat cold or hot! (Place the yogurt on the side if you want to eat the lamb balls hot, so then you don't have to heat the yogurt as well).

## *Smoked Salmon And Avocado Wholegrain Wraps*

**Total time:** 20 minutes

**Ingredients**

4 wholegrain wraps

2 cups lettuce, roughly sliced

2 avocadoes, flesh sliced

3 oz. smoked salmon

Olive oil

1 tbsp. balsamic vinegar mixed with 1 tablespoon of olive oil

**Directions**

Place your wraps onto a large board or clean bench.

Place a pile of lettuce onto each one, then add ½ an avocado (sliced) on top, place the salmon on top of the avocado and drizzle with olive oil and vinegar.

Carefully wrap your wraps into tight parcels, place into your containers and store in the fridge until needed.

## *Cold Tuna And Pasta Salad*

**Total time:** 30 minutes

**Ingredients**

1 ½ cups whole-meal penne pasta (or any other shapes you have handy!)

2 cans tuna (the single-serve cans) drained

2 carrots, peeled and cut into small pieces

¾ cup corn kernels

1 avocado, flesh cut into chunks

1 red bell pepper, core and seeds removed, flesh cut into small pieces

Salt and pepper, to taste

**Directions**

Bring a pot of water to boil and add pinch of salt and the dry pasta, cook until the pasta is al dente (some pastas differ so use the instructions on your packet).

Drain the pasta and leave to cool slightly before adding the tuna, carrots, corn, avocado, bell pepper, salt, pepper and a drizzle of olive oil.

Divide the pasta salad between your 4 containers, cover and place into the fridge to store until needed.

Serve cold!

## *Tuna, Corn, And Cheese Hot Sandwiches (For Cheat Days And Cravings)*

**Total time:** 15 minutes

**Ingredients**

4 slices of cheddar cheese

8 slices of wholegrain bread

1 cup corn kernels, fresh or canned

2 small cans of tuna (single-serve cans, half a can per sandwich)

Salt and pepper, to taste

**Directions**

Place a slice of cheese onto 4 of your bread slices, top with corn kernels and tuna, sprinkle with salt and pepper then place the other slice of bread on top of each sandwich.

Wrap in plastic wrap to keep the sandwiches together and place into your airtight containers.

Store in the fridge until need, and place into a hot sandwich press to toast before eating!

## *Stuffed Sweet Potatoes*

**Total time:** 20 minutes

**Ingredients**

4 sweet potatoes, pricked all over with a fork

1 scallion, finely chopped

Small handful of parsley, finely chopped

1 cup cottage cheese

1 cup baby spinach leaves

Salt and pepper, to taste

**Directions**

Place the sweet potatoes into the microwave and cook on HIGH for 1 minute increments until soft all the way through.

Cut the sweet potatoes in half and remove the flesh and place it into a small bowl.

Add the scallions, parsley, cottage cheese, spinach, salt and pepper, stir to combine.

Re-fill the sweet potato skins with the filling and place 2 halves into each of your 4 containers.

Place into the fridge to store until needed!

## *Grilled Chicken With Sweet Potatoes And Asparagus*

**Total time:** 35 minutes

**Ingredients**

4 small chicken breasts

1 large sweet potato, cut into chunks

16 spears of asparagus, tough ends removed

2 tbsp. olive oil

1 tsp. dried rosemary

Salt and pepper, to taste

**Directions**

Preheat the oven to 356 degrees Fahrenheit and prepare a tray by lining it with baking paper.

Place the chicken, sweet potato, asparagus, olive oil, rosemary, salt and pepper onto the tray and combine with your hands until everything is coated in oil and seasoning.

Place into the oven and bake for approximately 30 minutes or until the chicken is cooked through and the sweet potatoes are soft.

Divide between your 4 containers, cover, and place into the fridge until needed.

Eat hot or cold!

## *Brown Rice And Tuna Bowls*

**Total time:** 25 minutes

**Ingredients**

2 cups dry brown rice

4 small cans of unflavored tuna (the single-serve cans)

1 carrot, peeled and chopped into small pieces

1 red bell pepper, core and seeds removed, cut into small pieces

1 cup chopped cucumber

1 tbsp. balsamic vinegar

**Directions**

Place the brown rice into a pot and add 3 ½ cups of water and a pinch of salt, bring to the boil then reduce to a simmer, leave covered until the water has disappeared and the rice is soft (but still with a bite!).

Divide the cooked rice between your 4 containers and add the contents of one tuna can into each, divide the carrot, bell pepper, cucumber and balsamic vinegar between the 4 containers and stir to combine with the rice.

Cover and place into the fridge to store until needed!

# Chapter 8

# Dinner Meal Plan

## *Rainbow Chicken Salad*

**Total time:** 30 minutes

**Ingredients**

2 chicken breasts

Olive oil

Salt and pepper, to taste

½ head of red cabbage, thinly sliced

2 carrots, grated

1 cup cubed cucumber

2 yellow bell peppers, core and seeds removed, thinly sliced

½ head iceberg lettuce, roughly chopped

2 tomatoes, chopped into chunks

2 tbsp. balsamic vinegar mixed with 2 tbsp. olive oil

**Directions**

Preheat the oven to 356 degrees Fahrenheit and line a baking tray with baking paper.

Place the chicken breasts onto the tray and rub with olive oil, salt and pepper, place into the oven and bake for approximately 25 minutes or until cooked all the way through.

Slice the cooked chicken breasts into thin slices.

Place the cabbage, carrot, cucumber, bell peppers, lettuce, tomatoes, balsamic vinegar, olive oil and chicken into a large bowl and gently toss to combine and coat in oil and vinegar.

Divide the salad between your 6 containers, cover and place into the fridge to store until needed!

Eat within 3 nights of cooking (3 dinners for 2 people).

## *Veggie Stacks With Feta And Mint*

**Total time:** 25 minutes

**Ingredients**

8 large Portobello mushrooms

2 large zucchinis, sliced lengthways

1 large eggplant, sliced into 8 slices

2 large tomatoes, sliced

2 tbsp. olive oil

2 garlic cloves, crushed

Salt and pepper, to taste

3.5 oz. feta cheese

Small handful fresh mint leaves

**Directions**

Preheat the oven to 356 degrees Fahrenheit and line a baking tray with baking paper.

Lay the mushrooms, zucchini slices, eggplant slices, and tomato slices onto the tray and drizzle over the olive oil, garlic, salt and pepper.

Place the tray into the oven and bake for approximately 20 minutes until tender and golden.

Create your stacks by layering in this order: mushrooms, feta, zucchini slices, feta, eggplant slices, mint, tomato slices, feta, mint.

Place a skewer through the middle of each stack to keep them together if you like!

Pack away into your containers, cover and place into the fridge until needed.

## *Mexican-Inspired Shepherd's Pie*

**Total time:** 45 minutes

**Ingredients**

Olive oil

1 onion, finely chopped

17 oz. minced beef

2 cans (14 oz.) black beans, drained

1 tsp. chili powder

1 tsp. coriander

1 can (14 oz.) chopped tomatoes

2 large sweet potatoes, chopped into chunks

Salt and pepper, to taste

Large handful cilantro, roughly chopped

**Directions**

Preheat to oven to 356 degrees Fahrenheit.

Drizzle some olive oil into a large pot and place over a medium heat.

Place the onions into the pot and sauté until soft.

Add the minced beef and sauté until browned.

Add the black beans, chili powder, coriander and canned tomatoes, stir to combine.

Leave to simmer for about 10 minutes as you prepare the sweet potatoes.

Prick the sweet potatoes all over and place into the microwave, cook on HIGH for 1 minute increments until soft all the way through.

Cut the sweet potatoes into chunks and place into a bowl, mash with a potato masher or fork, add a pinch of salt and pepper and stir through.

Pour the mince and bean mixture into a large baking dish and spread the mashed sweet potatoes over top.

Sprinkle the coriander over the top of the sweet potatoes.

Place into the oven and bake for approximately 30 minutes until golden.

Leave to cool before cutting into 8 pieces, stacking into your airtight container/and store in the fridge or freezer until needed.

## *Swiss Chard And Ricotta Crust-Less Pie*

**Total time:** 30 minutes

**Ingredients**

Butter or cooking oil spray

5 eggs

9 oz. ricotta cheese

4 cups shredded Swiss chard

1 onion, finely chopped

½ cup grated cheddar cheese

Handful of fresh parsley, finely chopped

½tsp baking powder

Salt and pepper, to taste

**Directions**

Preheat the oven to 356 degrees Fahrenheit and grease a baking dish with butter or cooking oil spray.

Place all Ingredients, plus a pinch of salt and pepper into a bowl and whisk until fully combined.

Pour into your prepared baking dish and place into the oven.

Bake for approximately 25 minutes or until just set and beginning to turn golden on top.

Slice into 6 pieces, pack into your chosen containers cover and store in the fridge or freezer until needed!

A small drop of tomato relish goes really well on the side of this crust-less pie.

## *Steak And Zoodle Salad*

**Total time:** 25 minutes

**Ingredients**

3 large zucchinis, cut into noodles with a spiralizer

Saltand pepper, to taste

Olive oil

2 sirloin steaks (or 1 really large one, use your judgment to figure out how much steak you'd like for each serving)

Juice of one lemon mixed with 2 tbsp. olive oil

2 tbsp. sesame seeds

**Directions**

Place the zucchini noodles into a microwave-safe bowl and cook in the microwave for 1 minute. Don't overcook them, as you don't want them to be slushy or mushy! Sprinkle with salt and pepper and set aside.

Heat a small amount of olive oil in a non-stick frying pan and place over a high heat.

Place your steak onto the hot frying pan and cook to your liking, place onto a board to rest. You can season the steak with salt and pepper at this stage.

Keep the pan on the heat and add the sesame seeds to the pan and toast them in the leftover steak juices until golden and fragrant.

Thinly slice your steak and add to the bowl of zoodles, add the sesame seeds and the olive oil and lemon dressing, stir to combine.

Pack away into your container/s, cover and place into the fridge to store until needed!

I love to eat this salad cold, right out of the fridge.

## *Breaded Fish For The Freezer*

**Total time:** 15 minutes

**Ingredients**

2 eggs, lightly beaten

1 cup breadcrumbs mixed with a pinch of salt and pepper

4 large white fish filets, cut into 3 pieces each

**Directions**

Prepare by setting the working space with your beaten egg in a small bowl, and your breadcrumbs mixed with salt and pepper spread onto a plate, have your fish pieces next to them on a plate, ready to be dipped.

Have a tray lined with baking paper ready too, so you can put the coated fish on it to freeze.

Dip the fish pieces into the beaten eggs and transfer them straight into the breadcrumbs, turning to coat thoroughly on all sides.

Place the coated fish onto your lined tray, cover with plastic wrap and place into the freezer until almost frozen.

Place the almost-frozen fish pieces into your small container lined with baking paper, place another layer of paper between each layer of fish so they don't stick together.

Place straight into the oven from the freezer when you want to eat them! Don't thaw them out first.

## *Green Bean, Potato, And Pea Curry*

**Total time:** 30 minutes

**Ingredients**

Olive oil

4 garlic cloves, finely chopped

1 onion, finely chopped

4 tbsp. store-bought green curry paste

5 large potatoes, cut into cubes or chunks

2 cups frozen green beans

2 cups frozen peas

1 cup (8fl oz.) chicken or vegetable broth

3 cups (24fl oz.) coconut milk

Salt, to taste

**Directions**

Drizzle some olive oil into a large pot or pan and place over a medium heat.

Add the garlic, onions and curry paste, stir to combine and leave to sauté for a couple of minutes until the curry paste is fragrant.

Add the potatoes, beans, peas, broth and coconut milk to the pot and stir to combine, add a pinch of salt to season.

Allow the curry to boil for approximately 20 minutes or until the potatoes are soft but not mushy.

Leave to cool before dividing between your 6 containers, covering and placing into the fridge or freezer.

## *Coconut-Poached Fish With Peanuts And Asian Greens*

**Total time:** 25 minutes

**Ingredients**

1 ½ cups (12fl oz.) coconut milk

1 tsp. soy sauce

1 tsp. fish sauce

1 tsp. chili flakes

4 white fish filets

2 bunches of bok choi, base removed, leaves washed

½ cup roasted, salted peanuts

1 tsp. sesame oil

**Directions**

Add the coconut milk, soy sauce, fish sauce, chili flakes and fish filets into a deep fry pan or pot and place over a medium heat.

Bring to a gentle boil and leave to simmer for about 10 minutes or until the fish is just cooked.

Add the bok choi to the pot and place the lid onto the pot, leave for 1 minute to gently steam the bok choi.

Divide the fish, bok choi, and coconut milk between your 4 containers and sprinkle the peanuts and sesame oil over the top, cover and place into the fridge or freezer to store until needed.

If you like, a sprinkle of fresh chili and cilantro is a gorgeous addition before eating.

## *Marinated Steak Freezer Packets*

**Total time:** 15 minutes

**Ingredients**

4 beef steaks, cut into slices

2 tbsp. olive oil

2 tbsp. soy sauce

1 tbsp. honey

Salt and pepper, to taste

**Directions**

Place the steak strips, olive oil, soy sauce, honey, and a pinch of salt and pepper into a bowl and stir to combine, making sure each piece of beef is coated in oil, honey and sauce.

Divide the marinated steak between your 8 freezer-safe, sealable bags and stack into the freezer to store until needed.

To cook, leave to thaw in the bag before emptying into a hot frying pan to sauté with veggies, rice, egg or whatever you fancy!

## *Marinated Pork Packets*

**Total time:** 30 minutes

**Ingredients**

4 pork steaks, cut into slices

2 tbsp. olive oil

Juice of 1 lemon

1 small sprig of fresh rosemary, roughly chopped

1 tsp. dried mixed herbs (use fresh herbs if you have them, but don't worry if you don't, dried herbs are fine)

4 garlic cloves, crushed

**Directions**

**Place all Ingredients into a bowl and stir to combine, making sure the pork is thoroughly coated in oil, lemon juice, garlic and herbs.**

Divide between your 8 freezer-safe bags, seal and stack into the freezer to store until needed.

Leave to thaw before cooking in a hot frying pan.

## *Prepped Pasta Sauce: Tomato*

**Total time:** 30 minutes

**Ingredients**

Olive oil

6 garlic cloves, finely chopped

2 onions, finely chopped

3 cans (14 oz.) chopped tomatoes

2 tbsp. balsamic vinegar

1 tsp. honey

1 tsp. mixed dried herbs

Salt and pepper, to taste


**Directions**

Drizzle the olive oil into a frying pan and place over a medium heat.

Add the garlic and onions to the pan and sauté until soft.

Add the tomatoes, balsamic vinegar, honey, herbs, and a pinch of salt and pepper, stir to combine.

Cover the pot and leave to simmer on a low heat for 20 minutes.

## Ingredients

Olive oil

2 large salmon steaks, cut in half to make 4 even pieces

1 tbsp. soy sauce

1 tsp. sweet chili sauce

2 cups cooked brown lentils (I used canned ones, so much easier!)

1 ripe mango, skin removed, flesh cut into small chunks

4 fresh mint leaves, finely chopped

## Directions

Drizzle some olive oil into a non-stick fry pan and place over a medium heat.

Add the salmon pieces to the hot pan skin-side down and cook for 2 minutes on each side or until just cooked through.

Pour the soy sauce and chili sauce over the salmon.

Divide the lentils between your 4 containers, add the mango to each container, then place a piece of salmon on top, finish by sprinkling each pieces of salmon with the fresh mint.

Cover the containers and place into the fridge or freezer until needed!

# *Freezer Chicken Soup*

**Total time:** 30 minutes

**Ingredients**

5 boneless chicken thighs, cut into small pieces

1 onion, finely chopped

4 cups (32fl oz.) chicken broth

2 cups (16fl oz.) water

1 can (14 oz.) corn kernels, drained

2 scallions, finely sliced

Salt and pepper, to taste

**Directions**

Place all Ingredients into a pot and add a pinch of salt and pepper, place over a medium heat and cover.

Leave to simmer for approximately 30 minutes until the chicken is cooked through.

Leave to cool slightly before dividing into your 6 containers, cover and stack into the freezer to store until needed.

Leave the frozen containers on the bench to thaw before thoroughly reheating, or simply place the frozen soup in a pot over a high heat to speed the process up!

## *Prepped Pasta Sauce: Pesto*

**Total time:** 10 minutes

**Ingredients**

2 cups fresh basil leaves

3.5 oz. parmesan cheese, broken into small chunks

1/3 cup olive oil

3 garlic cloves, roughly chopped

½ cup pine nuts, (they are very expensive so just use cashew nuts for a cheaper option!)

Salt and pepper, to taste

**Directions**

Place all Ingredients into a blender or small food processor and add a pinch of salt and pepper.

Blend until smooth but still with a few small pieces of nuts remaining.

Pour into your jar or container and store in the fridge until needed!

You can also use this as a salad dressing for potato salads or chicken salads.

## *Prepped Pasta Sauce: Creamy Mushroom*

**Total time:** 20 minutes

## Ingredients

2 tbsp. olive oil

5 cups chopped mushrooms, (use a range of different kinds of mushrooms if you like! I use white button mushrooms and Portobello mushrooms)

8 garlic cloves, finely chopped

1 sprig of fresh rosemary, finely chopped

3fl oz. white wine

½ cup (4fl oz.) sour cream

½ cup (4fl oz.) plain yogurt

## Directions

Drizzle the olive oil into a frying pan and place over a medium heat.

Add the mushrooms, garlic and rosemary or mixed herbs, sauté for a few minutes until the mushrooms have begun to shrink and become colored.

Add the wine and simmer until the alcohol evaporates.

Add the sour cream and yoghurt and stir to combine.

Turn off the heat and leave the sauce to cool slightly before dividing into your 4 containers, cover and place into the freezer to store until needed!

# *Taco Freezer Packets*

**Total time:** 30 minutes

## Ingredients

3 large chicken breasts, cut into small slices

3 red bell peppers, core and seeds removed, thinly sliced

2 red onions, red onions, thinly sliced

2 cans (14 oz.) chopped tomatoes

6 garlic cloves, finely chopped

2 tsp. paprika

1 tsp. ground cumin

1 tsp. ground coriander

1 tsp. chili powder

2 tbsp. olive oil

## Directions

Place all Ingredients into a large bowl and stir to combine, making sure every piece of chicken and vegetables is coated in olive oil and spices.

Divide the mixture between your 8 freezer-safe sealable bags, seal and stack into the fridge to store until needed.

Leave to thaw before sautéing in a hot frying pan until cooked all the way through and the onions and bell peppers are slightly charred.

## *Breaded Chicken Freezer Packets*

**Total time:** 15 minutes

**Ingredients**

2 eggs, lightly beaten

2 cups breadcrumbs mixed with a pinch of salt and pepper

4 large chicken breasts, each cut into 6 pieces

**Directions**

Prepare your work space by placing the beaten egg in a small bowl next to a plate of breadcrumbs, salt and pepper.

Line a baking tray with baking paper and keep nearby so you can place your breaded chicken onto it.

Take your chicken pieces and dip them into the egg, then straight into the breadcrumbs, turning a few times to thoroughly coat in breadcrumbs.

Place the breaded chicken pieces onto your lined tray and place in the freezer.

Once frozen, divide the chicken pieces between your 8 freezer bags and stack into the freezer to store until needed!

To cook, simply preheat your oven to 356 degrees Fahrenheit, place the chicken pieces onto a lined baking tray and bake for about 25 minutes or until cooked through, no need to thaw first.

## *Stir-Fried Brown Rice With Chicken And Veggie Jewels*

**Total time:** 30 minutes

**Ingredients**

2 large chicken breasts

Olive oil

Salt and pepper

1 tsp. chili flakes

1 ½ cups dry brown rice

1 garlic clove, crushed

2 red bell peppers, core and seeds removed, cut into small pieces

2 scallions, finely chopped

8 spears of asparagus, cut into small pieces (the same size as the bell pepper pieces)

2 carrots, peeled and cut into pieces to match the asparagus and bell pepper pieces

2 tbsp. olive oil mixed with 1 tbsp. soy sauce

**Directions**

Preheat the oven to 356 degrees Fahrenheit and line a baking tray with baking paper.

Place the chicken breasts on the tray and drizzle with olive oil, salt, pepper and chili flakes, place into the oven for approximately 20 minutes or until the chicken is cooked through.

Leave the chicken to rest for a few minutes before cutting into small pieces.

Cook the rice while the chicken is cooking: place the brown rice into a pot and add 2 cups of water, place over a high heat and bring to the boil, reduce to a simmer and cook with the lid on until the water has disappeared and the rice is cooked.

Add the garlic, peppers, scallions, asparagus and carrot to the pot of rice and add the olive oil and soy sauce mixture, turn the heat up to high and keep stirring as the veggies cook in the rice – you can use a wok or fry pan for this step, but I just use the pot the rice cooked in to save myself another dish to wash up! It works perfectly well.

Add the chopped cooked chicken to the pot, stir through and leave to cool before dishing into your containers, cover and store in the fridge or freezer until needed!

## *Prepped Quinoa Sushi Rolls*

**Total time:** 25 minutes

**Ingredients**

1 cup quinoa

1 ½ cups water

14 oz. firm tofu, cut into strips

2 tbsp. soy sauce

1 tsp. sesame oil

1 tbsp. honey

6 nori sheets (sushi seaweed)

2 tbsp. sesame seeds, lightly toasted in a dry fry pan

1 red bell pepper, core and seeds removed, sliced

1 carrot, peeled and sliced into thin strips

**Directions**

Thoroughly rinse the quinoa in a sieve to remove the bitter outer layer.

Bring the water to the boil in a small pot and add the quinoa, stir to combine then turn the heat down to a simmer, cover, and cook for 12-15 minutes or until the liquid has disappeared and the quinoa is soft.

While the quinoa is cooking, prepare the tofu: place the soy sauce, sesame oil, honey and tofu into a small fry pan over a medium heat, cook for a few minutes until golden and cooked through, set aside.

Lay the nori sheets onto a large board, have your tofu, cooked quinoa, toasted sesame seeds and sliced veggies close by.

Spread a thin layer of quinoa onto each nori sheet, leaving an inch-wide gap at the top of each sheet.

Lay the tofu, carrot and bell peppers in a line in the center of the nori sheet (horizontally).

Sprinkle the sesame seeds on top of the tofu and veggies on each nori sheet.

Tightly roll the sushi and seal the ends with warm water.

Don't slice yet, wait until you're ready to eat to slice just before eating.

Pack the sushi rolls into your container and store in the fridge until needed!

## *Lamb And Red Onion Skewers*

**Total time:** 25 minutes

**Ingredients**

4 lamb leg steaks, cut into cubes

2 red onions, cut into 6 wedges each

2 tbsp. olive oil

Salt and pepper, to taste

8 skewers

**Directions**

Preheat the oven to 400 degrees Fahrenheit and line a baking tray with baking paper.

Load the skewers by alternating lamb and onion until full (but leave an inch on either side of the skewers so you can pick them up easily).

Rub the onion and lamb with olive oil and sprinkle with salt and pepper and place on the tray.

Place the tray into the oven and bake for approximately 20 minutes, turning once, until the onions are cooked and beginning to turn golden, and the lamb is cooked but still pink inside.

Leave the skewers to cool slightly before packing away into a large container, covering and storing in the fridge until needed.

## *Veggie Burgers Patties*

**Total time:** 25 minutes

**Ingredients**

5 Portobello mushrooms, cut into small pieces

1 cup corn kernels

1 cup chickpeas, drained and rinsed

2 eggs, lightly beaten

1 cup almond flour

Large handful of fresh parsley, finely chopped

1 tsp. ground cumin

1 tsp. ground coriander

1 tsp. chili powder

Salt and pepper, to taste

**Directions**

Preheat the oven to 356 degrees Fahrenheit and line a baking tray with baking paper.

**Place all Ingredients into a large bowl and add a pinch of salt and pepper.**

Vigorously stir until thoroughly combined.

Shape the mixture into 8 large patties.

Place the patties onto the baking tray and place into the oven.

Bake for about 7 minutes on each side (just take the tray out of the oven and turn the patties over after 7 minutes then put them back in for another 7) or until cooked through and golden on the outside.

Stack into an airtight container and store in the fridge until needed.

## *Freezer Soup (Pumpkin And Coconut)*

**Total time:** 45 minutes

## Ingredients

6 cups cubed pumpkin (skin removed, about 1 medium-sized pumpkin)

1 onion, finely chopped

2 carrots, cut into chunks

3 cups (24fl oz.) chicken stock

Salt and pepper, to taste

1 cup (8fl oz.) coconut milk

## Directions

Place the pumpkin, onion, carrots, stock, salt and pepper into a pot and bring to the boil, reduce to a simmer and simmer covered for about 25 minutes or until the veggies are soft.

Using a hand-held stick blender, blend until smooth.

Stir the coconut milk into the soup, taste, and add more salt and pepper if needed.

Allow it to cool slightly before pouring into your 6 containers, covering, then packing away into the freezer!

Remember to label the containers with masking tape and a sharpie so you can keep track of when the soup was made.

Simply take out of the freezer the morning of the day you want to have the soup for dinner, and leave to thaw on the kitchen bench.

Throw it into a pot or place into the microwave in a bowl to heat.

## *Spicy Lentil Stew With Sweet Potato Mash And Cilantro*

**Total time:** 40 minutes

**Ingredients**

Olive oil

1 onion, finely chopped

1 tsp. cumin

1 tsp. chili powder

1 tsp. ground coriander

1 can (14 oz.) chopped tomatoes

2 cans (14 oz.) brown lentils, drained

Salt and pepper, to taste

1 cup (8fl oz.) chicken stock

2 large sweet potatoes, cut into cubes

Large handful of cilantro, roughly chopped

**Directions**

Drizzle some olive oil into a pot and place over a medium heat.

Add the onion, cumin, chili, ground coriander, tomatoes, lentils, salt and pepper, stir to combine.

Add chicken stock to the pot.

Allow it to simmer for about 20 minutes until thick and rich.

As the lentil stew simmers, cook the sweet potatoes by pricking all over with a fork and cooking in the microwave on HIGH for 1 minute increments until soft all the way through.

Cut the cooked sweet potatoes into chunks and place into a bowl (I keep the skin on, it has nutrients!), add some salt and pepper and mash with a fork.

Divide the sweet potato mash between your 6 containers then divide the lentil stew between the containers and spoon on top of the sweet potatoes.

Sprinkle with fresh cilantro, cover and place into the fridge or freezer (or both, freeze 3, fridge 3!) until needed.

# Chapter 9

# Dessert Meal Plan

## *Fruit Kebab*

**Total time:** 30 minutes

**Ingredients**

3 apples

¼ cup orange juice

1 ½ lb. watermelon

¾ cup blueberries

Directions

Use a star-shaped cookie cutter to cut out stars from the apple and watermelon.

Soak the apple stars in orange juice.

Thread the apple stars, watermelon stars and blueberries into skewers.

Refrigerate for 30 minutes before serving.

## *Roasted Mangoes*

**Total time:** 15 minutes

## Ingredients

2 mangoes, peeled and sliced into cubes

2 tablespoons coconut flakes

2 teaspoons crystallized ginger, chopped

2 teaspoons orange zest

## Directions

Preheat your oven to 350 degrees F.

Put the mango cubes in custard cups.

Top with the ginger and orange zest.

Bake in the oven for 10 minutes.

# *Figs With Yogurt*

**Total time:** 8 hours 5 minutes

## Ingredients

8 oz. low fat yogurt

½ teaspoon vanilla

2 figs, sliced

1 tablespoon walnuts, toasted and chopped

Lemon zest

## Directions

Refrigerate yogurt in a bowl for 8 hours.

After 8 hours, take it out of the refrigerator and stir in yogurt and vanilla.

Stir in the figs.

Sprinkle walnuts and lemon zest on top before serving.

## *Strawberry & Watermelon Pops*

**Total time:** 6 hours 10 minutes

**Ingredients**

¾ cup strawberries, sliced

2 cups watermelon, cubed

¼ cup lime juice

2 tablespoons brown sugar

⅛ teaspoon salt

Directions

Put the strawberries inside popsicle molds.

In a blender, pulse the rest of the Ingredients until well mixed.

Pour the puree into a sieve before pouring into the molds.

Freeze for 6 hours.

# *Cinnamon Almond Balls*

**Total time:** 15 minutes

**Ingredients**

1 tsp cinnamon

3 tbsp erythritol

1 ¼ cup almond flour

1 cup peanut butter

Pinch of salt

**Directions:**

Add all Ingredients into the mixing bowl and mix well.

Cover and place bowl in fridge for 30 minutes.

Make small bite size ball from mixture and serve.

# *Choco Frosty*

**Total time:** 10 minutes

**Ingredients**

1 tsp vanilla

8 drops liquid stevia

2 tbsp unsweetened cocoa powder

1 tbsp almond butter

1 cup heavy cream

**Directions:**

Add all Ingredients into the mixing bowl and beat with immersion blender until soft peaks form.

Place in refrigerator for 30 minutes.

Add frosty mixture into the piping bag and pipe in serving glasses.

Serve and enjoy.

## *Moist Avocado Brownies*

**Total time:** 45 minutes

**Ingredients**

2 avocados, mashed

2 eggs

1 tsp baking powder

2 tbsp swerve

1/3 cup chocolate chips, melted

4 tbsp coconut oil, melted

2/3 cup unsweetened cocoa powder

**Directions:**

Preheat the oven to 325 F.

In a mixing bowl, mix together all dry Ingredients.

In another bowl, mix together avocado and eggs until well combined.

Slowly add dry mixture to the wet along with melted chocolate and coconut oil. Mix well.

Pour batter in greased baking pan and bake for 30-35 minutes.

Slice and serve.

## *Mix Berry Sorbet*

**Total time:** 0 minutes

**Ingredients**

½ cup raspberries, frozen

½ cup blackberries, frozen

1 tsp liquid stevia

6 tbsp water

**Directions:**

Add all Ingredients into the blender and blend until smooth.

Pour blended mixture into the container and place in refrigerator until harden.

Serve chilled and enjoy.

## *Chia Almond Pudding*

**Total time:** 10 minutes

## Ingredients

2 tbsp almonds, toasted and crushed

1/3 cup chia seeds

½ tsp vanilla

4 tbsp erythritol

¼ cup unsweetened cocoa powder

2 cups unsweetened almond milk

## Directions:

Add almond milk, vanilla, sweetener, and cocoa powder into the blender and blend until well combined.

Pour blended mixture into the bowl.

Add chia seeds and whisk for 1-2 minutes.

Pour pudding mixture into the serving bowls and place in fridge for 1-2 hours.

Top with crushed almonds and serve.

# *Choco Peanut Cookies*

**Total time:** 20 minutes

## Ingredients

1 cup peanut butter

1 tsp baking soda

2 tsp vanilla

1 tbsp butter, melted

2 eggs

2 tbsp unsweetened cocoa powder

2/3 cup erythritol

1 1/3 cups almond flour

**Directions:**

Preheat the oven to 350 F.

Add all Ingredients into the mixing bowl and stir to combine.

Make 2-inch balls from mixture and place on greased baking tray and gently press down each ball with fork.

Bake in oven for 8-10 minutes.

Serve and enjoy.

## *Chocolate Macaroon*

**Total time:** 30 minutes

**Ingredients**

1 tsp vanilla

¼ cup coconut oil

2 eggs

1/3 cup unsweetened coconut, shredded

1/3 cup erythritol

½ tsp baking powder

¼ cup unsweetened cocoa powder

3 tbsp coconut flour

1 cup almond flour

Pinch of salt

**Directions:**

Add all Ingredients into the mixing bowl and mix until well combined.

Make small balls from mixture and place on greased baking tray.

Bake at 350 F for 15-20 minutes.

Serve and enjoy.

## *Mocha Ice-Cream*

**Total time:** 20 minutes

**Ingredients**

¼ tsp xanthan gum

1 tbsp instant coffee

2 tbsp unsweetened cocoa powder

15 drops liquid stevia

2 tbsp erythritol

¼ cup heavy cream

1 cup unsweetened coconut milk

**Directions:**

Add all Ingredients except xanthan gum into the blender and blend until smooth.

Add xanthan gum and blend until mixture is slightly thickened.

Pour mixture into the ice cream maker and churn according to machine instructions.

Serve chilled and enjoy.

## *Fruit Salad*

**Total time:** 10 minutes

**Ingredients**

1 tsp erythritol

1 tsp lemon juice

1 sage leaf, chopped

1 tbsp blueberries

¼ cup strawberries, sliced

½ cup raspberries

½ cup blackberries

**Directions:**

Add all Ingredients into the bowl and toss well.

Serve and enjoy.

## *Blackberry Pops*

**Total time:** 20 minutes

**Ingredients**

1 tsp liquid stevia

½ cup water

1 fresh sage leaf

1 cup blackberries

**Directions:**

Add all Ingredients into the blender and blend until smooth.

Pour blended mixture into the ice pop molds and place in refrigerator for overnight.

Serve and enjoy.

## *Peanut Butter Banana Splits*

**Total time:** 10 minutes

**Ingredients:**

6 bananas, sliced

2 tablespoons coconut oil

4 tablespoons peanut butter

1 cup chocolate chips

To serve:

Non Dairy whipped topping

Non Dairy frozen treats

Maraschino cherries

Strawberry slices

**Directions:**

Add chocolate chips, coconut oil, and peanut butter into a microwave-safe bowl. Microwave on high for about a minute. Whisk well. If the mixture is not melted, place for a few more seconds. Whisk after every 5 seconds.

Divide the banana slices into 6 glasses or bowls.

Drizzle the chocolate sauce over the bananas. Refrigerate until use. It can last for 2 days.

To serve: Remove the glasses from the refrigerator. Top with the suggested toppings and serve.

## *Apple Strudel*

**Total time:** 20 minutes

**Ingredients:**

2 packages vegan puff pastry dough (16 x 9 inches each)

1 ½ teaspoons ground cinnamon

4 red apples, peeled, cored, cut into thin slices using a slicer

Powdered vegan sugar, to sprinkle (optional)

**Directions:**

Sprinkle cinnamon over the apple and stir using your hands.

Unfold the pastry dough on your countertop. Place apple slices on one half of the dough. Fold the other half over the filling. Press the edges to seal. Place in an airtight container in the refrigerator. It can last for 2 days.

To serve: Bake in a preheated oven at 350° F for 15 – 20 minutes or until brown on top.

Serve warm or at room temperature.

## *Pumpkin Parfaits*

**Total time:** 10 minutes

**Ingredients:**

4 cups vanilla soy yogurt

½ cup brown or raw sugar (optional)

½ teaspoon ground nutmeg

2 cups pumpkin puree

1 teaspoon ground cinnamon

¼ teaspoon ground ginger (optional)

**Topping:**

4 squares dark chocolate, melted

8 ginger snap cookies, broken

Mint leaves

**Directions:**

Add pumpkin, yogurt, sugar, ginger, cinnamon, and nutmeg into a bowl and whisk until sugar dissolves completely.

Divide into glasses. Refrigerate until use. It can last for 3 days.

To serve: Top with the suggested toppings and serve.

## *Peanut Butter Balls*

**Total time:** 10 minutes

**Ingredients:**

1/3 cup roasted peanuts

1 tablespoon cocoa powder

3 tablespoons rolled oats

½ cup pitted Medjool dates

**Directions:**

Add dates into the food processor and pulse until smooth.

Add rest of the Ingredients and pulse until well combined.

Divide the mixture into 8 equal portions and shape into balls. Place in an airtight container and refrigerate until use. It can last for a week.

To freeze: Place in freezer-safe bags and freeze until use. It can last for 2 months.

## *Fig, Coconut, And Blackberry Ice Cream*

**Total time:** 6 hours 20 minutes

**Ingredients:**

20 fresh, ripe figs, chop each into 8 pieces

Juice of a lemon

Zest of a lemon, grated

4 teaspoons ginger, minced (optional)

4 cups coconut milk

1 1/3 cups blackberries + extra to garnish

¾ cup water

2/3 cup dried shredded coconut, unsweetened

1 cup agave nectar or to taste

A few leaves lemon balm

**Directions:**

Place a saucepan over medium heat. Add figs, water, lemon zest, dried coconut, and ginger. When it begins to boil, lower the heat and simmer until figs are tender.

Add blackberries and agave nectar and cook until slightly thick.

Turn off the heat and cool completely. Blend with an immersion blender until smooth.

Add rest of the Ingredients and blend for a few seconds until the fruits get chopped into tiny pieces. Pour into a bowl. Cover and chill for 4 – 6 hours.

Pour into an ice cream maker and churn the ice cream following the manufacturer's instructions. Transfer into a freezer-safe container. Freeze until use.

To serve: Remove from the freezer and place for 10 minutes on your countertop before serving. Scoop ice cream into bowls. Serve garnished with blackberries and lemon balm.

## *Layered Blueberry Cheesecake*

**Total time:** 1 hour 10 minutes

**Ingredients:**

For crust:

1 cup almond flour

1 cup raw pecans

6 dates, pitted

2 teaspoons ground cinnamon

4 tablespoons coconut oil

½ teaspoon kosher salt

For filling:

4 cups raw cashew, soaked in water for 4-8 hours

½ cup coconut oil, melted, cooled

4 tablespoons fresh lemon juice

½ cup freeze-dried blueberries

½ cup canned coconut milk, shake the can well before pouring into the cup

2/3 cup pure maple syrup

2 tablespoons vanilla extract or 1 teaspoon vanilla bean powder

For blueberry layer:

2 cups blueberries, fresh or frozen, thawed if frozen

2 tablespoons chia seeds

2 tablespoons fresh lemon juice

## Directions:

Grease 2 small springform pans with coconut oil. Place strips of parchment paper in it.

Add all the Ingredients of crust into the food processor and pulse until well combined and slightly sticky. Do not pulse for long.

Divide the mixture into the prepared pans. Press it well into the bottom of the pan.

To make filling: Add all the Ingredients for filling into the food processor and pulse until smooth. Add more coconut milk if the mixture is not getting smooth while blending. Taste and adjust sweetness if desired. Set aside about 1/3 of the filling and add into a bowl. Add freeze-dried blueberries and mix well. Set aside.

Divide the remaining 2/3 of the filling in the 2 crusts. Spread it evenly.

Freeze for an hour.

Divide the blueberry mixture on top of both the crusts. Place the cheesecakes in the freezer.

To make blueberry layer: Add all the Ingredients for blueberry layer into the blender and blend until smooth.

Pour on the top of the crusts. Place the cheesecakes back in the freezer. Freeze until firm. It can last for a week.

Serve frozen or thawed. Cut into wedges and serve.

## *Chocolate Fudge Cookies*

**Total time:** 30 minutes

**Ingredients:**

2 large ripe bananas, sliced

1 cup peanut butter or any other nut butter of your choice

Flaky sea salt to sprinkle

1 cup cocoa powder

1 cup + 2 tablespoons maple syrup

**Directions:**

Add banana into a bowl. Using a fork, mash the bananas.

Stir in peanut butter, maple syrup and cocoa powder. Mix until well combined.

Place a sheet of parchment paper on 1 – 2 large baking sheets. Place tablespoonful of the mixture at different spots. You should have about 28 cookies in all.

Bake in a preheated oven at 325° F for 15 minutes. Remove from the oven and sprinkle salt over the cookies. Let it cool to room temperature. Transfer into an airtight container. It can last for 10 – 12 days.

# *Apple Pie*

**Total time:** 90 minutes

**Ingredients:**

For the crust:

½ cup + 1 tablespoon all-purpose flour

3 tablespoons organic vegan shortening, cut into small cubes

1/8 teaspoon salt

2 tablespoons ice water

For the filling:

¼ teaspoon ground cinnamon

½ tablespoon lemon juice

½ tablespoon cornstarch

¼ cup packed light brown sugar

For topping:

¼ cup rolled oats

1 ½ tablespoons packed light brown sugar

1 tablespoon organic vegan shortening

2 tablespoons all-purpose flour

¼ teaspoon ground cinnamon

**Directions:**

To make crust: Add flour into a bowl. Add cold shortening. Cut it into the flour using a pastry cutter until crumbs are formed.

Add ice-cold water, a tablespoon at a time and mix until a moist dough is formed.

Shape into a circle of about 4-5 inches.

Take a sheet of plastic wrap. Sprinkle some flour on it. Place the dough in the middle of the sheet and wrap it completely. Place in the refrigerator for a maximum of 2 days.

Remove from the refrigerator 15 minutes before preparing.

To make the filling: Add apples, brown sugar, cinnamon and lemon juice into a bowl. Mix well and set aside for 15 minutes.

Sprinkle cornstarch and toss until well coated.

Place a sheet of parchment paper on your countertop. Place dough on the center of the parchment paper. Cover with another sheet of parchment paper. Roll with a rolling pin until about 6 – 7 inches in diameter. Carefully remove the top parchment paper.

Lift the dough along with the bottom parchment paper, carefully invert onto a 5 – 6-inch pie pan. Press the dough into the pan.

Carefully remove the other parchment paper.

Place the filling in the pie pan. Spread it all over the pan.

Bake in a preheated oven at 375°F for 15-20 minutes.

To make the topping: Add all the Ingredients of the topping into a bowl. Cut it into the flour using a pastry blender or a pair of knives until smaller pieces are formed.

Then use your hands and mix until the mixture is crumbly. Sprinkle over the apple filling in the pie.

Bake for 30-40 minutes until the top is golden brown. It can last for 2 – 3 days. Place in an airtight container at room temperature.

Cut into wedges and serve.

## *Salted Caramel Chocolate Cups*

**Total time:** 10 minutes

**Ingredients:**

½ cup dark chocolate chips

3 tablespoons vegan caramel sauce

1 teaspoon coconut oil

1/8 teaspoon flaky sea salt

**Directions:**

Place disposable cupcake liners in a 6 counts muffin pan.

Add chocolate chips and coconut oil into a microwave-safe bowl. Microwave on high for about 50 seconds. Whisk well. If the mixture is not melted, place for a few more seconds. Whisk after every 5 seconds.

Divide most of the chocolate mixture among the cupcake liners. Using the back of a spoon, spread it evenly on the bottom as well as a little on the sides of the liners.

Freeze until firm. Divide the caramel sauce among the cupcake liners. Drizzle the remaining chocolate on the caramel layer.

Refrigerate until use. It can last for a week.

## *Creamy Mint Chocolate Chip Avocado Ice Cream*

**Total time:** 50 minutes

**Ingredients:**

4 medium-large Hass avocados, peeled, pitted, chopped into chunks

½ cup coconut butter or coconut oil

2 tablespoons peppermint extract

½ cup chocolate chips

2 medium bananas, peeled, sliced

4 tablespoons maple syrup or coconut nectar or agave nectar

15-20 fresh mint leaves (optional)

**Directions:**

Add all the Ingredients except chocolate chips into a blender and blend until smooth.

Pour into a freezer-safe container. Freeze for an hour.

Remove the ice cream from the freezer and whisk well. Refreeze and beat again after 30-40 minutes.

Repeat the previous step 2 – 3 times until well frozen without ice crystals.

Add chocolate chips and stir when you whisk for the last time.

## *Quick Mug Brownie*

**Total time:** 6 minutes

**Ingredients**

2 eggs

1 tbsp heavy cream

1 scoop protein powder

1 tbsp erythritol

¼ tsp vanilla

**Directions:**

Add all Ingredients into the mug and mix well.

Place mug in microwave and microwave for 1 minute.

Serve and enjoy.

## *Protein Peanut Butter Ice Cream*

**Total time:** 10 minutes

**Ingredients**

5 drops liquid stevia

2 tbsp heavy cream

2 tbsp peanut butter

2 tbsp protein powder

¾ cup cottage cheese

**Directions:**

Add all Ingredients into the blender and blend until smooth.

Pour blended mixture into the container and place in refrigerator for 30 minutes.

Serve chilled and enjoy.

## *Chia Raspberry Pudding*

**Total time:** 10 minutes

**Ingredients**

¼ tsp vanilla

¾ cup unsweetened almond milk

1 tbsp erythritol

2 tbsp proteins collagen peptides

¼ cup chia seeds

½ cup raspberries, mashed

**Directions:**

Add all Ingredients into the bowl and stir until well combined.

Place in refrigerator for overnight.

Serve chilled and enjoy.


## *Chocolate Chia Pudding*

**Total time:** 30 minutes

**Ingredients**

½ cup chia seeds

½ tsp vanilla

1/3 cup unsweetened cocoa powder

1 ½ cups unsweetened coconut milk

**Directions:**

Add all Ingredients into the mixing bowl and whisk well.

Place bowl in refrigerator for overnight.

Serve chilled and enjoy.

## *Cheesecake Fat Bombs*

**Total time:** 20 minutes

**Ingredients**

8 oz cream cheese

1 ½ tsp vanilla

2 tbsp erythritol

4 oz coconut oil

4 oz heavy cream

**Directions:**

**Add all Ingredients into the mixing bowl and beat using immersion blender until creamy.**

Pour batter into the mini cupcake liner and place in refrigerator until set.

Serve and enjoy.

## *Matcha Ice Cream*

**Total time:** 1030 minutes

**Ingredients**

½ tsp vanilla

2 tbsp swerve

1 tsp matcha powder

1 cup heavy whipping cream

**Directions:**

Add all Ingredients into the glass jar.

Seal jar with lid and shake for 4-5 minutes until mixture double.

Place in refrigerator for 3-4 hours.

Serve chilled and enjoy.

## *Grilled Peaches*

**Total time:** 8 minutes

**Ingredients**

1 cup balsamic vinegar

⅛ teaspoon ground cinnamon

1 tablespoon honey

3 peaches, pitted and sliced in half

2 teaspoons olive oil

6 gingersnaps, crushed

**Directions**

Pour the vinegar into a saucepan.

Bring it to a boil.

Lower heat and simmer for 10 minutes.

Remove from the stove.

Stir in cinnamon and honey.

Coat the peaches with oil.

Grill peaches for 2 to 3 minutes.

Drizzle each one with syrup.

Top with the gingersnaps.

## *Fruit Salad*

**Total time:** 5 minutes

**Ingredients**

8 oz. light cream cheese

6 oz. Greek yogurt

1 tablespoon honey

1 teaspoon orange zest

1 teaspoon lemon zest

1 orange, sliced into sections

3 kiwi fruit, peeled and sliced

1 mango, cubed

1 cup blueberries

**Directions**

Beat cream cheese using an electric mixer.

Add yogurt and honey.

Beat until smooth.

Stir in the orange and lemon zest.

Toss the fruits to mix.

Divide in glass jars.

Top with the cream cheese mixture.

## *Choco Banana Bites*

**Total time:** 2 hours 10 minutes

**Ingredients**

2 bananas, sliced into rounds

¼ cup dark chocolate cubes

**Directions**

Melt chocolate in the microwave or in a saucepan over medium heat.

Coat each banana slice with melted chocolate.

Place on a metal pan.

Freeze for 2 hours.

# *Blueberries With Yogurt*

**Total time:** 5 minutes

**Ingredients**

1 cup nonfat Greek yogurt

¼ cup blueberries

¼ cup almonds

**Directions**

Add yogurt and blueberries in a food processor.

Pulse until smooth.

Top with almonds before serving.

# *Chocolate & Raspberry Ice Cream*

**Total time:** 12 hours 20 minutes

**Ingredients**

¼ cup almond milk

2 egg yolks

2 tablespoons cornstarch

¼ cup honey

¼ teaspoon almond extract

⅛ teaspoon salt

1 cup fresh raspberries

2 oz. dark chocolate, chopped

¼ cup almonds, slivered and toasted

**Directions**

Mix almond milk, egg yolks, cornstarch and honey in a bowl.

Pour into a saucepan over medium heat.

Cook for 8 minutes.

Strain through a sieve.

Stir in salt and almond extract.

Chill for 8 hours.

Put into an ice cream maker.

Follow manufacturer's directions.

Stir in the rest of the Ingredients.

Freeze for 4 hours.

# *Mocha Pops*

**Total time:** 4 minutes

**Ingredients**

3 cups brewed coffee

½ cup low calorie chocolate flavored syrup

¾ cup low fat half and half

**Directions**

Mix the Ingredients in a bowl.

Pour into popsicle molds.

Freeze for 4 hours.

# Chapter 10

# Snack Meal Plan

## *Crab Dip*

Preparation time: 10 minutes

Cooking time: 30 minutes

Servings: 8

**Ingredients:**

bacon strips, sliced

ounces crab meat

½ cup mayonnaise

½ cup sour cream

ounces cream cheese

poblano pepper, chopped

tablespoons lemon juice

Salt and black pepper to the taste

garlic cloves, minced

green onions, minced

½ cup parmesan cheese+ ½ cup parmesan cheese, grated

Salt and black pepper to the taste

**Directions:**

Heat up a pan over medium high heat, add bacon, cook until it's crispy, transfer to paper towels, chop and leave aside to cool down.

In a bowl, mix sour cream with cream cheese and mayo and stir well.

Add ½ cup parmesan, poblano peppers, bacon, green onion, garlic and lemon juice and stir again.

Add crab meat, salt and pepper and stir gently.

Pour this into a heat proof baking dish, spread the rest of the parmesan, introduce in the oven and bake at 350 degrees F for 20 minutes.

Serve your dip warm with cucumber stick.

Enjoy!

**Nutrition Value:**

calories 200, fat 7, fiber 2, carbs 4, protein 6

## *Simple Spinach Balls*

Preparation time: 10 minutes

Cooking time: 12 minutes

Servings: 30

## Ingredients:

tablespoons melted ghee

eggs

1 cup almond flour

16 ounces spinach

1/3 cup feta cheese, crumbled

¼ teaspoon nutmeg, ground

1/3 cup parmesan, grated

Salt and black pepper to the taste

1 tablespoon onion powder

tablespoons whipping cream

1 teaspoon garlic powder

## Directions:

In your blender, mix spinach with ghee, eggs, almond flour, feta cheese, parmesan, nutmeg, whipping cream, salt, pepper, onion and garlic pepper and blend very well.

Transfer to a bowl and keep in the freezer for 10 minutes

Shape 30 spinach balls, arrange on a lined baking sheet, introduce in the oven at 350 degrees F and bake for 12 minutes.

Leave spinach balls to cool down and serve as a party appetizer.

Enjoy!

**Nutrition Value:**

calories 60, fat 5, fiber 1, carbs 0.7, protein 2

# *Garlic Spinach Dip*

Preparation time: 10 minutes

Cooking time: 35 minutes

Servings: 6

**Ingredients:**

bacon slices

ounces spinach

½ cup sour cream

ounces cream cheese, soft

1 and ½ tablespoons parsley, chopped

ounces parmesan, grated

1 tablespoon lemon juice

Salt and black pepper to the taste

1 tablespoon garlic, minced

**Directions:**

Heat up a pan over medium heat, add bacon, cook until it's crispy, transfer to paper towels, drain grease, crumble and leave aside in a bowl.

Heat up the same pan with the bacon grease over medium heat, add spinach, stir, cook for 2 minutes and transfer to a bowl.

In another bowl, mix cream cheese with garlic, salt, pepper, sour cream and parsley and stir well.

Add bacon and stir again.

Add lemon juice and spinach and stir everything.

Add parmesan and stir again.

Divide this into ramekins, introduce in the oven at 350 degrees f and bake for 25 minutes.

Turn oven to broil and broil for 4 minutes more.

Serve with crackers.

Enjoy!

**Nutrition Value:**

calories 345, fat 12, fiber 3, carbs 6, protein 11

## *Mushrooms Appetizer*

Preparation time: 10 minutes

Cooking time: 20 minutes

Servings: 5

**Ingredients:**

¼ cup mayo

1 teaspoon garlic powder

1 small yellow onion, chopped

24 ounces white mushroom caps

Salt and black pepper to the taste

1 teaspoon curry powder

ounces cream cheese, soft

¼ cup sour cream

½ cup Mexican cheese, shredded

1 cup shrimp, cooked, peeled, deveined and chopped

**Directions:**

In a bowl, mix mayo with garlic powder, onion, curry powder, cream cheese, sour cream, Mexican cheese, shrimp, salt and pepper to the taste and whisk well.

Stuff mushrooms with this mix, place on a baking sheet and cook in the oven at 350 degrees F for 20 minutes.

Arrange on a platter and serve.

Enjoy!

**Nutrition Value:**

calories 244, fat 20, fiber 3, carbs 7, protein 14

## *Simple Bread Sticks*

Preparation time: 10 minutes

Cooking time: 15 minutes

Servings: 24

**Ingredients:**

tablespoons cream cheese, soft

1 tablespoon psyllium powder

¾ cup almond flour

cups mozzarella cheese, melted for 30 seconds in the microwave

1 teaspoon baking powder

1 egg

tablespoons Italian seasoning

Salt and black pepper to the taste

ounces cheddar cheese, grated

1 teaspoon onion powder

**Directions:**

In a bowl, mix psyllium powder with almond flour, baking powder, salt and pepper and whisk.

Add cream cheese, melted mozzarella and egg and stir using your hands until you obtain a dough.

Spread this on a baking sheet and cut into 24 sticks.

Sprinkle onion powder and Italian seasoning over them.

Top with cheddar cheese, introduce in the oven at 350 degrees F and bake for 15 minutes.

Serve them as a keto snack!

Enjoy!

**Nutrition Value:**

calories 245, fat 12, fiber 5, carbs 3, protein 14

## *Italian Meatballs*

Preparation time: 10 minutes

Cooking time: 6 minutes

Servings: 16

**Ingredients:**

1 egg

Salt and black pepper to the taste

¼ cup almond flour

1 pound turkey meat, ground

½ teaspoon garlic powder

tablespoons sun dried tomatoes, chopped

½ cup mozzarella cheese, shredded

tablespoons olive oil

tablespoon basil, chopped

**Directions:**

In a bowl, mix turkey with salt, pepper, egg, almond flour, garlic powder, sun dried tomatoes, mozzarella and basil and stir well.

Shape 12 meatballs, heat up a pan with the oil over medium high heat, drop meatballs and cook them for 2 minutes on each side.

Arrange on a platter and serve.

Enjoy!

**Nutrition Value:**

calories 80, fat 6, fiber 3, carbs 5, protein 7

## *Parmesan Wings*

Preparation time: 10 minutes

Cooking time: 24 minutes

Servings: 6

**Ingredients:**

pound chicken wings, cut in halves

Salt and black pepper to the taste

½ teaspoon Italian seasoning

tablespoons ghee

½ cup parmesan cheese, grated

A pinch of red pepper flakes, crushed

1 teaspoon garlic powder

1 egg

## Directions:

Arrange chicken wings on a lined baking sheet, introduce in the oven at 425 degrees F and bake for 17 minutes.

Meanwhile, in your blender, mix ghee with cheese, egg, salt, pepper, pepper flakes, garlic powder and Italian seasoning and blend very well.

Take chicken wings out of the oven, flip them, turn oven to broil and broil them for 5 minutes more.

Take chicken pieces out of the oven again, pour sauce over them, toss to coat well and broil for 1 minute more.

Serve them as a quick keto appetizer.

Enjoy!

## Nutrition Value:

calories 134, fat 8, fiber 1, carbs 0.5, protein 14

## *Cheese Sticks*

Preparation time: 1 hour and 10 minutes

Cooking time: 20 minutes

Servings: 16

**Ingredients:**

eggs, whisked

Salt and black pepper to the taste

mozzarella cheese strings, cut in halves

1 cup parmesan, grated

1 tablespoon Italian seasoning

½ cup olive oil

1 garlic clove, minced

**Directions:**

In a bowl, mix parmesan with salt, pepper, Italian seasoning and garlic and stir well.

Put whisked eggs in another bowl.

Dip mozzarella sticks in egg mixture, then in cheese mix.

Dip them again in egg and in the parmesan mix and keep them in the freezer for 1 hour.

Heat up a pan with the oil over medium high heat, add cheese sticks, fry them until they are golden on one side, flip and cook them the same way on the other side.

Arrange them on a platter and serve.

Enjoy!

**Nutrition Value:**

calories 140, fat 5, fiber 1, carbs 3, protein 4

## *Tasty Broccoli Sticks*

Preparation time: 10 minutes

Cooking time: 20 minutes

Servings: 20

**Ingredients:**

1 egg

cups broccoli florets

1/3 cup cheddar cheese, grated

¼ cup yellow onion, chopped

1/3 cup panko breadcrumbs

1/3 cup Italian breadcrumbs

tablespoons parsley, chopped

A drizzle of olive oil

Salt and black pepper to the taste

**Directions:**

Heat up a pot with water over medium heat, add broccoli, steam for 1 minute, drain, chop and put into a bowl.

Add egg, cheddar cheese, panko and Italian breadcrumbs, salt, pepper and parsley and stir everything well.

Shape sticks out of this mix using your hands and place them on a baking sheet which you've greased with some olive oil.

Introduce in the oven at 400 degrees F and bake for 20 minutes.

Arrange on a platter and serve.

Enjoy!

**Nutrition Value:**

calories 100, fat 4, fiber 2, carbs 7, protein 7

# *Bacon Delight*

Preparation time: 15 minutes

Cooking time: 1 hour and 20 minutes

Servings: 16

**Ingredients:**

½ teaspoon cinnamon, ground

tablespoons erythritol

16 bacon slices

1 tablespoon coconut oil

ounces dark chocolate

1 teaspoon maple extract

**Directions:**

In a bowl, mix cinnamon with erythritol and stir.

Arrange bacon slices on a lined baking sheet and sprinkle cinnamon mix over them.

Flip bacon slices and sprinkle cinnamon mix over them again.

Introduce in the oven at 275 degrees F and bake for 1 hour.

Heat up a pot with the oil over medium heat, add chocolate and stir until it melts.

Add maple extract, stir, take off heat and leave aside to cool down a bit.

Take bacon strips out of the oven, leave them to cool down, dip each in chocolate mix, place them on a parchment paper and leave them to cool down completely.

Serve cold.

ioy!

**ꞁ Value:**

ꞁt 4, fiber 0.4, carbs 1.1, protein 3

# *Taco Cups*

Preparation time: 10 minutes

Cooking time: 40 minutes

Servings: 30

**Ingredients:**

1 pound beef, ground

cups cheddar cheese, shredded

¼ cup water

Salt and black pepper to the taste

tablespoons cumin

tablespoons chili powder

Pico de gallo for serving

**Directions:**

Divide spoonfuls of parmesan on a lined baking sheet, introduce in the oven at 350 degrees F and bake for 7 minutes.

Leave cheese to cool down for 1 minute, transfer them to mini cupcake molds and shape them into cups.

Meanwhile, heat up a pan over medium high heat, add beef, stir and cook until it browns.

Add the water, salt, pepper, cumin and chili powder, stir and cook for 5 minutes more.

Divide into cheese cups, top with pico de gallo, transfer them all to a platter and serve.

Enjoy!

**Nutrition Value: calories 140, fat 6, fiber 0, carbs 6, protein 15**

## *Tasty Chicken Egg Rolls*

Preparation time: 2 hours and 10 minutes

Cooking time: 15 minutes

Servings: 12

**Ingredients:**

ounces blue cheese

cups chicken, cooked and finely chopped

Salt and black pepper to the taste

green onions, chopped

celery stalks, finely chopped

½ cup tomato sauce

½ teaspoon erythritol

egg roll wrappers

Vegetable oil

## Directions:

In a bowl, mix chicken meat with blue cheese, salt, pepper, green onions, celery, tomato sauce and sweetener, stir well and keep in the fridge for 2 hours.

Place egg wrappers on a working surface, divide chicken mix on them, roll and seal edges.

Heat up a pan with vegetable oil over medium high heat, add egg rolls, cook until they are golden, flip and cook on the other side as well.

Arrange on a platter and serve them.

Enjoy!

## Nutrition Value:

calories 220, fat 7, fiber 2, carbs 6, protein 10

# *Halloumi Cheese Fries*

Preparation time: 10 minutes

Cooking time: 5 minutes

Servings: 4

**Ingredients:**

1 cup marinara sauce

ounces halloumi cheese, pat dried and sliced into fries

ounces tallow

**Directions:**

Heat up a pan with the tallow over medium high heat.

Add halloumi pieces, cover, cook for 2 minutes on each side and transfer to paper towels.

Drain excess grease, transfer them to a bowl and serve with marinara sauce on the side.

Enjoy!

**Nutrition Value:**

calories 200, fat 16, fiber 1, carbs 1, protein 13

## *Jalapeno Crisps*

Preparation time: 10 minutes

Cooking time: 25 minutes

Servings: 20

**Ingredients:**

tablespoons olive oil

jalapenos, sliced

ounces parmesan cheese, grated

½ teaspoon onion powder

Salt and black pepper to the taste

Tabasco sauce for serving

**Directions:**

In a bowl, mix jalapeno slices with salt, pepper, oil and onion powder, toss to coat and spread on a lined baking sheet.

Introduce in the oven at 450 degrees F and bake for 15 minutes.

Take jalapeno slices out of the oven, leave them to cool down.

In a bowl, mix pepper slices with the cheese and press well.

Arrange all slices on a another lined baking sheet, introduce in the oven again and bake for 10 minutes more.

Leave jalapenos to cool down, arrange on a plate and serve with Tabasco sauce on the side.

Enjoy!

**Nutrition Value:**

calories 50, fat 3, fiber 0.1, carbs 0.3, protein 2

## *Delicious Cucumber Cups*

Preparation time: 10 minutes

Cooking time: 0 minutes

Servings: 24

**Ingredients:**

cucumbers, peeled, cut in ¾ inch slices and some of the seeds scooped out

½ cup sour cream

Salt and white pepper to the taste

ounces smoked salmon, flaked

1/3 cup cilantro, chopped

teaspoons lime juice

1 tablespoon lime zest

A pinch of cayenne pepper

**Directions:**

In a bowl mix salmon with salt, pepper, cayenne, sour cream, lime juice and zest and cilantro and stir well.

Fill each cucumber cup with this salmon mix, arrange on a platter and serve as a keto appetizer.

Enjoy!

**Nutrition Value:**

calories 30, fat 11, fiber 1, carbs 1, protein 2

# *Caviar Salad*

Preparation time: 6 minutes

Cooking time: 0 minutes

Servings: 16

**Ingredients:**

eggs, hard boiled, peeled and mashed with a fork

ounces black caviar

ounces red caviar

Salt and black pepper to the taste

1 yellow onion, finely chopped

¾ cup mayonnaise

Some toast baguette slices for serving

**Directions:**

In a bowl, mix mashed eggs with mayo, salt, pepper and onion and stir well.

Spread eggs salad on toasted baguette slices, and top each with caviar.

Enjoy!

**Nutrition Value:**

calories 122, fat 8, fiber 1, carbs 4, protein 7

# *Marinated Kebabs*

Preparation time: 20 minutes

Cooking time: 10 minutes

Servings: 6

**Ingredients:**

1 red bell pepper, cut in chunks

1 green bell pepper, cut into chunks

1 orange bell pepper, cut into chunks

pounds sirloin steak, cut into medium cubes

garlic cloves, minced

1 red onion, cut into chunks

Salt and black pepper to the taste

tablespoons Dijon mustard

and ½ tablespoons Worcestershire sauce

¼ cup tamari sauce

¼ cup lemon juice

½ cup olive oil

**Directions:**

In a bowl, mix Worcestershire sauce with salt, pepper, garlic, mustard, tamari, lemon juice and oil and whisk very well.

Add beef, bell peppers and onion chunks to this mix, toss to coat and leave aside for a few minutes.

Arrange bell pepper, meat cubes and onion chunks on skewers alternating colors, place them on your preheated grill over medium high heat, cook for 5 minutes on each side, transfer to a platter and serve as a summer keto appetizer.

Enjoy!

**Nutrition Value:**

calories 246, fat 12, fiber 1, carbs 4, protein 26

## *Simple Zucchini Rolls*

Preparation time: 10 minutes

Cooking time: 5 minutes

Servings: 24

**Ingredients:**

tablespoons olive oil

zucchinis, thinly sliced

24 basil leaves

tablespoons mint, chopped

1 and 1/3 cup ricotta cheese

Salt and black pepper to the taste

¼ cup basil, chopped

Tomato sauce for serving

**Directions:**

Brush zucchini slices with the olive oil, season with salt and pepper on both sides, place them on preheated grill over medium heat, cook them for 2 minutes, flip and cook for another 2 minutes.

Place zucchini slices on a plate and leave aside for now.

In a bowl, mix ricotta with chopped basil, mint, salt and pepper and stir well.

Spread this over zucchini slices, divide whole basil leaves as well, roll and serve as an appetizer with some tomato sauce on the side.

Enjoy!

**Nutrition Value:**

calories 40, fat 3, fiber 0.3, carbs 1, protein 2

## *Simple Green Crackers*

Preparation time: 10 minutes

Cooking time: 24 hours

Servings: 6

## Ingredients:

cups flax seed, ground

cups flax seed, soaked overnight and drained

bunches kale, chopped

1 bunch basil, chopped

½ bunch celery, chopped

garlic cloves, minced

1/3 cup olive oil

## Directions:

In your food processor mix ground flaxseed with celery, kale, basil and garlic and blend well.

Add oil and soaked flaxseed and blend again.

Spread this into a tray, cut into medium crackers, introduce in your dehydrator and dry for 24 hours at 115 degrees F, turning them halfway.

Arrange them on a platter and serve.

Enjoy!

## Nutrition Value:

calories 100, fat 1, fiber 2, carbs 1, protein 4

## *Cheese And Pesto Terrine*

Preparation time: 30 minutes

Cooking time: 0 minutes

Servings: 10

**Ingredients:**

½ cup heavy cream

ounces goat cheese, crumbled

tablespoons basil pesto

Salt and black pepper to the taste

sun dried tomatoes, chopped

¼ cup pine nuts, toasted and chopped

1 tablespoons pine nuts, toasted and chopped

**Directions:**

In a bowl, mix goat cheese with the heavy cream, salt and pepper and stir using your mixer.

Spoon half of this mix into a lined bowl and spread.

Add pesto on top and also spread.

Add another layer of cheese, then add sun dried tomatoes and ¼ cup pine nuts.

Spread one last layer of cheese and top with 1 tablespoon pine nuts.

Keep in the fridge for a while, turn upside down on a plate and serve.

Enjoy!

**Nutrition Value:**

calories 240, fat 12, fiber 3, carbs 5, protein 12

## *Avocado Salsa*

Preparation time: 10 minutes

Cooking time: 0 minutes

Servings: 4

**Ingredients:**

1 small red onion, chopped

avocados, pitted, peeled and chopped

jalapeno pepper, chopped

Salt and black pepper to the taste

tablespoons cumin powder

tablespoons lime juice

½ tomato, chopped

**Directions:**

In a bowl, mix onion with avocados, peppers, salt, black pepper, cumin, lime juice and tomato pieces and stir well.

Transfer this to a bowl and serve with toasted baguette slices as a keto appetizer.

Enjoy!

**Nutrition Value:**

calories 120, fat 2, fiber 2, carbs 0.4, protein 4

## *Tasty Egg Chips*

Preparation time: 5 minutes

Cooking time: 10 minutes

Servings: 2

**Ingredients:**

½ tablespoon water

tablespoons parmesan, shredded

eggs whites

Salt and black pepper to the taste

**Directions:**

In a bowl, mix egg whites with salt, pepper and water and whisk well.

Spoon this into a muffin pan, sprinkle cheese on top, introduce in the oven at 400 degrees F and bake for 15 minutes.

Transfer egg white chips to a platter and serve with a keto dip on the side.

Enjoy!

**Nutrition Value:**

calories 120, fat 2, fiber 1, carbs 2, protein 7

## *Chili Lime Chips*

Preparation time: 10 minutes

Cooking time: 20 minutes

Servings: 4

**Ingredients:**

1 cup almond flour

Salt and black pepper to the taste

1 and ½ teaspoons lime zest

1 teaspoon lime juice

1 egg

**Directions:**

In a bowl, mix almond flour with lime zest, lime juice and salt and stir.

Add egg and whisk well again.

Divide this into 4 parts, roll each into a ball and then spread well using a rolling pin.

Cut each into 6 triangles, place them all on a lined baking sheet, introduce in the oven at 350 degrees F and bake for 20 minutes.

Enjoy!

**Nutrition Value:**

calories 90, fat 1, fiber 1, carbs 0.6, protein 3

## *Artichoke Dip*

Preparation time: 10 minutes

Cooking time: 15 minutes

Servings: 16

**Ingredients:**

¼ cup sour cream

¼ cup heavy cream

¼ cup mayonnaise

¼ cup shallot, chopped

1 tablespoon olive oil

garlic cloves, minced

ounces cream cheese

½ cup parmesan cheese, grated

1 cup mozzarella cheese, shredded

ounces feta cheese, crumbled

1 tablespoon balsamic vinegar

28 ounces canned artichoke hearts, chopped

Salt and black pepper to the taste

ounces spinach, chopped

**Directions:**

Heat up a pan with the oil over medium heat, add shallot and garlic, stir and cook for 3 minutes.

Add heavy cream and cream cheese and stir.

Also add sour cream, parmesan, mayo, feta cheese and mozzarella cheese, stir and reduce heat.

Add artichoke, spinach, salt, pepper and vinegar, stir well, take off heat and transfer to a bowl.

Serve as a tasty keto dip.

Enjoy!

**Nutrition Value:**

calories 144, fat 12, fiber 2, carbs 5, protein 5

# *Baked Parsley Cheese Fingers*

Preparation Time: 15 minutes

Servings: 2-4

**Ingredients**

1 cup pork rinds, crushed

1 egg

1 tbsp dried parsley

1 lb cheddar cheese, cut into sticks

**Directions**

Preheat oven to 350 F and line a baking sheet with parchment paper. Combine pork rinds and parsley in a bowl to be evenly mixed. Beat the egg in another bowl.

Coat the cheese sticks in the egg and then generously dredge in pork rind mixture. Arrange on the baking sheet. Bake for 4 to 5 minutes, take out after, let cool for 2 minutes, and serve with marinara sauce.

**Nutrition Value:**

Calories: 213, Fat: 19.5g, Net Carbs: 1.5g, Protein: 8.7g

# Conclusion

Once you get the hang of meal prepping you will never want to go back! Having packets of fresh, healthy food packed away in the fridge and freezer, ready to be eaten is a satisfying and gratifying feeling. If these recipes do not quite fit in with your particular weight-loss diet, then simply modify them until the macronutrients are where you want them to be! Less carbs? No worries. More protein? Easy. Just download a calorie-counting app, load the recipes in, and shuffle things around to reach your desired numbers.

Always remember to prep meals that you **want to eat!** In my opinion, the best foods are healthy **and** delicious, and once you hit that sweet-spot you can lose weight without even noticing that you've changed your diet! You'll be so satisfied and full from your yummy, nutrient-filled foods that you won't get that horrible sense of deprivation and craving which comes with many strict diets.

Make a day of it and go shopping for containers, oils, spices, non-perishables, masking tape and sharpies for labeling, a diary to plan your meals and prep days, and put it all in a pretty and space-saving box.

Make your prep-sessions fun and relaxing, as they should be! You deserve to enjoy your life, your diet, and your kitchen.
Good luck and have fun!

CPSIA information can be obtained
at www.ICGtesting.com
Printed in the USA
BVHW041204180221
600497BV00006B/281

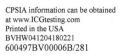

9 781914 251870